"We are all caregivers at some point in our lives, but taking care of a loved one is often not openly discussed. This remarkable book dares to be honest and raw about caring for a loved one with dementia. Compassion, frustration, tears, patience, impatience, acceptance, guilt—*Taming the Chaos of Dementia* explores the full range of emotions experienced by both those with dementia as well as those providing the care. The authors detail the exhaustive emotions that run in a circle while you grieve the loss of a person you once knew. There is only the present moment a caregiver gets to see, a glimpse, a hug, a tear, a touch, and hope for a brief glimmer of recognition. This amazing, empathetic, book covers not only the experiences through personal stories but provides evidence-based insights and solutions to help all caregivers cope with the process of caring for a loved one with dementia, or "our person" as so poignantly referenced in this book. This is a book for everyone to read—it sparks the humanity in all of us."

— **Jane Rohde, AIA, FIIDA, ASID, CHID, ACHA, EDAC, principal of JSR Associates, Inc. and founder of Live Together, Inc.**

"*Taming the Chaos of Dementia* brings valuable insight in how dementia induced behaviors of anxiety and confusion can be moderated with simple home environment interventions like color, sound, light, and sensory engagement. For caregivers seeking to practice creative approaches to enrich the lives of those journeying with dementia while caring for self, this book provides an insightful path for practical problem solving."

— **Ruth Shea, OFS, MSW, LICSW, geriatric social worker**

"Despite billions in research dollars and numerous promises of pharmacologic cures that keep Wall Street buzzing—the "silver bullet" to relieve society of dementia and its burdens eludes us. Barbara Huelat has seen dementia as a family member, care giver, designer, and esearcher. Few even approach her level of experience and perspective on living with dementia. But beyond that breadth of experience, expertise, research, and knowledge is a profound human hand in all the insights, pearls, hacks, and advice. That steady human touch guiding the application of science and experience is really needed to 'Tame the Chaos.' Huelat and Pochron have been able to accumulate, assemble, and present what is known scientifically and combine that with touching and real human experiences so that we can apply knowledge to challenges of dementia. Spoiler alert! The reader may well end up with more insight into dementia care than several of the healthcare providers they will encounter in their journey. "

— **Mik Pietzrak**

"Huelat and Pochron liken being a personal caregiver for someone who has dementia to being like Alice finding herself in a disturbing new Wonderland after tumbling down a rabbit hole. Even more troubling is the reality that the size and gravitational pull of that rabbit hole will continue to exponentially increase as the baby boom generation ages into old age. In the absence of a cure or prevention for dementia, therapeutic interventions, including supportive home design features, have the potential to offer the most wide-ranging treatment opportunities to people around the globe. The need for sensitively designed home environments that support resilience in people and their caregivers is becoming critically important. Barbara Huelat, in particular, tackles this topic with the same research-oriented attention to detail as she has in her design work for the last five decades, providing the next generation of caregivers with practical tools and advice on how to leverage design to thrive in a complex situation."

— **Debra Levin, Hon. FASID, EDAC, president and CEO of The Center for Health Design**

Taming the Chaos of Dementia

A Caregiver's Guide to Interventions That Make a Difference

BARBARA J. HUELAT AND
SHARON T. POCHRON, PHD

ROWMAN & LITTLEFIELD
Lanham • Boulder • New York • London

Published by Rowman & Littlefield
An imprint of The Rowman & Littlefield Publishing Group, Inc.
4501 Forbes Boulevard, Suite 200, Lanham, Maryland 20706
www.rowman.com

86-90 Paul Street, London EC2A 4NE

British Library Cataloguing in Publication Information Available

Library of Congress Cataloging-in-Publication Data

Names: Huelat, Barbara J., author. | Pochron, Sharon T., author.
Title: Taming the chaos of dementia : a caregiver's guide to interventions that make a difference / Barbara J. Huelat and Sharon T. Pochron, PhD.
Description: Lanham : Rowman & Littlefield, [2023] | Includes bibliographical references and index.
Identifiers: LCCN 2023022046 (print) | LCCN 2023022047 (ebook) | ISBN 9781538178980 (cloth) | ISBN 9781538178997 (ebook)
Subjects: LCSH: Dementia—Popular works. | Dementia—Patients—Care—Popular works. | Dementia—Patients—Family relationships. | Alzheimer's disease—Popular works. | Alzheimer's disease—Patients—Care—Popular works. | Alzheimer's disease—Patients—Family relationships.
Classification: LCC RC521 .H834 2023 (print) | LCC RC521 (ebook) | DDC 616.8/31—dc23/eng/20230703
LC record available at https://lccn.loc.gov/2023022046
LC ebook record available at https://lccn.loc.gov/2023022047

In loving memory of
Maxcine, Clara, Joseph Sr.,
and by my beloved Joe,
for allowing me to share in their
dementia journey.

Contents

Acknowledgments

I am so grateful to my loved ones, especially my mom, Maxcine, my grandmother, Clara, my father-in-law, Joseph Sr., and my dear husband and soul mate, Joe, for their great wisdom and for sharing their journey into the depths of dementia. Without them, this book could not exist. I sincerely appreciate my family, especially Vicky, my sister-in-law, my brothers, Bruce Huelat, Jerry, Larry, Brian, and Guy, along with their wives and children, for each contributing their tender caregiving support of mom and assistance to me. Deep gratitude to my daughters, Sharon Pochron and Julie Pochron, who continually provided counsel, listening hearts, and sound advice through caregiving and the writing of this book. A special thank-you to Sharon for patiently editing and guiding me through the writing and publishing process. Most prominently, Sharon has transformed this professional content into a readable and delightful work. A special thanks to Grace Boateng for her beautiful drawings that grace this book and Mark Murphy, who rescued my lost files, and his IT support.

I wish to express my appreciation to all the caregivers I interviewed, sharing their personal stories. A special thank-you to Joanne Newton, Jon Wiant, Jennifer Tilghman, Melani Swartz, and Clevis Laird, who were kind enough to allow me video interviews. I thank my numerous dear friends for their encouragement, listening, patience, and suggestions, especially

Abbot Joseph, Father Elias, Mother Theodora, Angela Tilghman, Clara Tucker, Peter Brooks, Shelly and Jim Whitmeire, Dana Oprisan, MD, Wayne Ruga, and Cate Kinney.

I would like to thank all my healthcare and design colleagues for my dementia education, especially Michael Pietrzak, MD, for his visionary human approach to dementia design and the honor to work with him on his multiple memory care facilities throughout the country. I am genuinely thankful to Ying-Chyi Chou, PhD, for the extraordinary opportunity to work with her at Tunghai University and for urging me to write this important book. I am also grateful to Thomas Wan, PhD, for his research support and counsel in geriatrics, aging, and technology, as well as his introduction to geriatric needs in Taiwan. Finally, a big thank-you and much appreciation to Rowman & Littlefield for taking on this important book.

Preface

BARBARA'S PREFACE

This book has a back story starting in my childhood. In my little brown Girl Scout uniform, my ten-year-old self walked through what seemed like a warehouse of old people. We sang Christmas carols and distributed our meager handmade gifts to an endless row of elderly people confined to their beds at Oak Forest Infirmary. The sadness and hopelessness haunted me then and haunts me still. As a child I wondered, "Is this what happens to people when they get old?" As an adult, I still wonder, "How can we improve their lives and the lives of the people who love them?"

The eyes—some haunted, some empty—drove me to my profession of healthcare design and to my desire to create healing environments. Over the next fifty years, those eyes were still in my mind as I discovered the ways in which design interventions were both possible and beautiful. When my loved ones started aging, my journey became more poignant. I had to start practicing the tools I'd brought to others, refining them in the process. Surviving the heart attack caused by that journey brought me great insight, and all the pieces came together for me. I realized that caregivers had access to the emotions of their people with dementia, and that access was possible via not only design but via activities—and love. I wish I'd had this book when I was caring for my people.

The Oak Forest image is still present in my mind, but I find it diminished. By finding new and creative ways to honor and share our love with our people with dementia, I feel like maybe I've done right by all those haunted eyes. As you read this book, I wish you hope and patience. Whether you're reading this early or late in your journey with your person, I can personally assure you that you still have happiness ahead of you.

—Barbara J. Huelat, January 2023

SHARON'S PREFACE

I began working with my mom on this book as an act of love. I had the skills she needed: I teach a course on epidemiology at Stony Brook University, I had coauthored a peer-reviewed article on the topic of dementia and the caregiver with my mom, and I had written many, many research papers on topics tangential to this one. My mom ached with desire to write this book, and I could help her meet a life goal.

I took on this project because I love my mom, but I was super crabby about it. Writing a book is hard. As a professor with grants, teaching, research, and service, I didn't have a lot of time for her project. Every minute I spent editing and researching was time away from my own research.

I don't think I appreciated the beauty of this project until we began to revise the chapter on music. Part of my job in the writing of this book required that I fact-check mom's ideas by reading the peer-reviewed literature. When we got to the music section, I realized that not only can scientists verify that we can reach the minds of people with dementia via music, but we know why. I took a step back at that moment—we were three-quarters of the way through the manuscript—and I realized that scientists could verify all of the tools my mom had collected in this book. And furthermore, she'd taken those ideas and applied them in her own life. I had a moment when I sat back and thought to myself, "Wow. This book really is going to help a lot of people stay connected with their person while taking care of themselves." My mom is amazing.

I'm sure glad this project was foisted upon me. My crabbiness has been replaced with gratitude and respect. I hope you find this book as amazing as I do.

—Sharon T. Pochron, PhD, January 2023

Introduction

Environmental Interventions for Dementia

Before you can move in new directions, you must first let go of what's not working for you.

—*Alberto Villoldo*

Following gall bladder surgery, Joe, with mid-stage Alzheimer's disease, required a six-week stay at a rehab nursing home. Our little dog and I would visit daily and cheer his spirits. It was a beautiful summer afternoon, but the nursing home felt oppressive. We needed an outing. I secured the wheelchair, and then Joe, our dog, and I set off for a neighborhood stroll. It began as a delightful walk, and we enjoyed the summer flowers and trees. Then I began to feel the strain as I pushed his wheelchair over the uneven pavement, the cracks in the sidewalk, and the curbs. The sidewalk sloped downward, and I quickened to keep pace with the gravity-fed wheelchair. The slope steepened, and I was now at a slow run. I was starting to feel out of control and needed to stop but could not. Now nearing a run, the handle grips on the wheelchair came loose in my hands, and I started running full speed to catch up, but Joe careened down the hill. Finally, I threw myself in front of the chair just before we crashed. We were terribly shaken, and I was bruised and emotionally traumatized.

Back at home, I contemplated the near disaster of my afternoon, and it struck me how analogous my fateful wheelchair adventure was to the dementia journey. Much like my walk, the journey starts with love, empathy, and good intentions. As the disease progresses, the journey gets bumpier and rougher. You find you must change strategy to keep up, you start to feel out of control, you lose your grip, and finally it's out of your hands. You throw yourself into the impending disaster as a last resort. And I wondered: Is this the obligatory journey, or is there a better way?

MEET THE WOLF

My mother used to call it old-timer's disease. She wasn't sure if it was just getting old or if there was more to it. Either way, dementia lurks out there, and as we age, we hope it won't be the wolf on our personal doorstep. When we can't remember a name or misplace our keys, quiet fear bites our secret hearts. It happens to your neighbor, your bridge partner, that gentleman in the grocery store. Last week you discussed your vacation with your dear friend, and this week he struggles with your name. We try to play it light. "There's something not right about my mom. She's outside at midnight picking the neighbor's flowers but says she just wanted to surprise me," a friend said. Our neighbors and friends don't look any different. She still has her characteristic giggle, and he still yells at traffic. But then, one day, it happens. The police call because he went to the post office, didn't remember where he lived, and couldn't find his way home. Then the trip to the doctor, the test, more tests, and the diagnosis. It looks like dementia, most likely Alzheimer's disease. It's the verdict that one in ten people over sixty-five will get it.[1]

My mom had Parkinson's disease with dementia. She hallucinated spiders creeping down her shirt and a family living in her basement. My father-in-law had dementia from Alzheimer's disease and confused the sink for the toilet. My grandmother had a stroke, which confused her timeframe, and she wanted to plant her tomatoes in January. And finally, I lost my dear friend and husband to Alzheimer's disease and learned to understand the disease on a very human level.

I have lived with them, laughed with them, cried with them, solved problems with them, and journeyed through the long, confusing path from the first diagnosis, to adapting their home, to moving from house to care facilities, and then to their eventual passing. Caregiving is not an easy journey, regardless of the empathy and love you share with them. It is an emotional journey and visceral experience of learning, research, sadness, and joy while untangling symptoms from triggers and behaviors and finding pieces of life that truly bring joy to their life and your own.

When the wolf came to my door, I drew on my years of professional experiences in planning and designing senior living environments, as well as personal relationships. I sought guidance from counselors, physicians, clients, other professionals, and resources, which was a daunting task. Yet when each of my loved ones passed, they left a big hole. I missed them and wondered if I did the right things. Could I have handled that meltdown better? Could I have brought more happiness into their lives? When my best friend, partner, and husband passed, I investigated how other caregivers managed. Did they have tools that I didn't know? My investigation led to research projects and presentations that I shared with Planetree, universities, clients, and other organizations. It led me to write this book and share what I have learned, hoping it makes other people's journeys with these diseases a little less challenging.

I have learned you can sometimes change adverse outcomes, minimize meltdowns, and engage with people with dementia in nonverbal communication. There are ways to keep them smiling and reduce caregiver stress. I don't have a magic bullet to share. I have no cure, and my interventions don't work all the time. But the interventions offered here can help improve the quality of life for those living with dementia and reduce the caregiver's burden of stress. I offer simple, inexpensive tools that work at the emotional and visceral levels. Most of these interventions have research and evidence behind them; others require greater study.

Dementia is a complex, confusing, and uniquely personal illness. My late father-in-law suffered from Alzheimer's, as did my husband; my grandmother was afflicted with vascular dementia because of several mini strokes, my mother battled Parkinson's disease. These various pathologies generated cognitive impairments, yet each response was surprisingly similar—each person communicated through emotions, not cognitive skills.

Each of my loved ones taught me critical lessons that I would like to share. I learned to read their body language, their pleasures, joys, pain, and frustrations, their reactions to situations and places they found themselves in. Each person with their unique personality tried to communicate the best they knew how, and sometimes that communication felt desperate. These experiences have also enabled me to apply these lessons. I watched my husband's and loved ones' cognitive skills decline, yet their emotional, intuitive side remained intact and often took over for their lack of cognitive abilities. I learned to communicate with their emotions.

DEMENTIA: WHAT IS IT?

Dementia isn't a specific disease. It's a broad term describing all types of diseases and illnesses affecting memory and cognitive processing. It affects our ability to solve problems and remember people and places. It robs our minds while leaving our physical body relatively intact. Every type of dementia has one thing in common: a loss of intellectual or cognitive ability.

Of the disease that presents as dementia, Alzheimer's disease is the most common. In fact, 50 to 77 percent of dementia is linked to Alzheimer's disease. Other common types of dementia include vascular dementia, Lewy body dementia, and frontotemporal dementia. Dementia can also occur as part of Parkinson's disease, syphilis, normal pressure hydrocephalus, Creutzfeldt-Jakob disease, and many more. Some dementias are linked to prescription medications, especially in combination with each other. Dementia affected about 46 million people in 2015. It is the most common disability among the elderly and is estimated to cost $604 billion annually.

The World Health Organization labels dementia a global public health priority. Many nations are developing dedicated plans for providing adequate care and support for both people with dementia and their caregivers.[2] Care solutions frequently focus on empowering people with dementia to live better and safer at home. Governmental dementia care plans frequently rely on innovative assistive technology and an increased emphasis on the potential volunteer support commitment.[3] We must consider the options to effectively manage this population's needs.

Healthcare professionals often refer to the "phases" or "stages" of dementia, describing how far the disease has progressed in an individual. The early stage is mild and often not detectable except by close relatives. During the middle or moderate phase, the disease might be detectable by others, but people in this stage can still function with a bit of support. During the severe or late phases, people with dementia may fully lose their ability to communicate via traditional methods. For clinical use, these phases may be subdivided into stages or scales closely associated with symptoms or behaviors that change over time and phase.[4]

Sufferers of dementia will differ in their care needs from the initial diagnosis through the duration of the disease. Individuals may not require care assistance at the initial diagnosis, but that need will change as the disease progresses. Therefore, activities and interventions must change to accommodate the person's physical and cognitive ability to participate. Some interventions are helpful at all phases, such as sensory interventions, music therapy, and biophilic interventions; other interventions, such as games and puzzles or movement therapies requiring motor skills, are most appropriate in early or mid-phases.[5]

People in early-stage dementia can function independently but may need reminders of names and tasks. At this phase, active interventions should remain independent. Caregivers can focus on maintaining social relationships, hobbies, and activities. During the middle phase, a decline in cognitive skills will become noticeable, and the individual loses some independence as assistance with daily living is required. During this phase, interventions can significantly help bridge the gap between emotional need and behavior. Late-stage dementia will require significant care as the person with dementia becomes fully dependent on the caregiver. Most individuals in this stage cannot perform activities of daily living or move independently. Don't give up hope for people in the late stage. Most therapies and interventions presented in this book have modified applications for those living within the late phase of dementia.

WHY INTERVENTION MATTERS

We know that dementia sufferers will gradually lose memory, learning ability, and an understanding of how things work. As dementia continues, their conditions worsen, and they are less able to care of themselves. We care for our loved ones; we keep them safe; we take away their car keys and place them in safe homes with other people with this disabling condition. In the struggle to do the right thing, we often make assumptions about what is best—and seclude them from joy and meaning.

Do people with dementia have any insight into their declining condition? Do they experience joy, excitement, sadness, grief, anger, and distress? Science shows that as dementia sufferers lose their cognitive functions, they do not lose their ability to enjoy life, love and be loved, laugh, cry, and connect with relationships.[6]

However, dementia sufferers have emotional problems and lack filters, leading to uninhibited behaviors. This creates great difficulty caring for those with dementia. The emotional portion of the brain learns through societal influences. We know from a young age how to act and control inappropriate behaviors. However, as the cognitive abilities decline, the ability to manage emotions also declines, depriving the person living with dementia of a socially acceptable response. Unfortunately, disruptive behaviors and meltdowns by people with dementia often lead to restraints, sedative medications, and physical conflict with others.[7]

This book will discuss multiple interventions that can help bridge the emotional experience with sensory, perceptive, and reminiscent memory to help mitigate disruptive behaviors and their triggers. Interventions do not stop dementia but can significantly increase the quality of life for those with dementia and their caregivers. It can transform the care of those with dementia from merely keeping them safe to providing a rich experience. Our brains use two memory systems: episodic and semantic memory. Episodic memory includes life events or autobiographical memory. Semantic memory holds abstract knowledge such as concepts, facts, and vocabulary.[8] While people with dementia experience loss in both areas, semantic memory and short-term memory are more significantly disrupted. Emotions are closely associated with episodic memory, personal events, and personal experiences. Effective interventions lean into the autobiographical sensory memory and increase links between experience and memory.

My longtime design client and noted trauma physician Dr. Michael Pietrzak explained the science behind memory and the design for dementia care environments. "There is a general acceptance and substantiation that memories connected with very emotional events are more unforgettable. They always say, 'You never forget your first . . .' All those highly emotional events tend to occur at ages sixteen through twenty-eight—first kiss, first love, first marriage, hanging out with friends, wild parties, etc. Thus, my premise is to include the icons of memory around those ages of the clients."

Research has shown how emotional autobiographical memories of past events can be stimulated through the individual use of various interventions tied to undamaged parts of the brain.[9] My work with Dr. Pietrzak in the design of memory care facilities, as well as my personal experiences in caregiving, have led me to explore this exciting possibility. Many dementia caregivers have seen that linking memory, sensory perception, and reflection with place can improve the quality of life. It can change behavioral outcomes.[10] This book offers interventions that lean into the emotional memories to engage your loved one even in the late stages of dementia, while taking care of yourself.

*   *   *

If you've ever cared for someone with dementia, you might empathize with Alice, who tumbled down a rabbit hole and discovered herself in an unhappy world where time moved oddly and animals and plants spoke, mostly to berate you. Familiar objects became terribly out of scale. If you're caring for someone with dementia now, you might feel like someone changed the rules of reality and that you need a guide, preferably someone kinder than the perennially late rabbit.

This book supports the journey—taken by both the caregiver and the person with dementia—providing loved ones with practical recommendations based on evidence and enriched with human empathy. Recommendations help ease the burden of stress by offering interventions and non-pharmaceutical therapeutic suggestions. They help decode dementia's visceral world and support noncognitive human experiences.

This book offers real stories from the journeys of authentic people who have struggled to survive the chaos and challenges driven by dementia. I've paired these accounts with practical examples of interventions that target the miseries of disruptive behaviors, environmental triggers, and factors that induce them.

Suggested interventions are evidence based and explore options in human engagement, the experience of destinations, positive distractions, familiar settings, furnishings, light, color, technology, nature, and the emotion of the senses. This book shows how interventions really can support the family caregivers in functional and emotional outcomes.

I survived three challenging years of dementia caregiving, further surviving a heart attack, stress, sleepless nights, and being overwhelmed with caregiving tasks; I asked myself, "Do all caregivers of dementia go through similar journeys? Do they need to?" I am suggesting we consider adding human-centric interventions as powerful tools to improve the quality of life for people with dementia. This is the journey I share with you.

The Art of Caregiving

> Care is a state in which something does matter; it is the source of human tenderness.
>
> —Rollo May

I found myself alone and scared, lying on a gurney in the emergency room. Joe was home, waiting for me without his day caregiver. What had happened? I recall returning from a difficult out-of-town business trip earlier that evening. I had sent Joe's caregiver home and was making dinner. Then I had that pain again in my chest that I couldn't explain. I called the triage nurse, and she told me to come in immediately, so I drove myself to the Emergency Department and left Joe, saying, "I will be home shortly." But that didn't happen. After a whirlwind of activities and tests, the doctors concluded that I'd had a heart attack.

I couldn't believe it. I was too busy for a heart attack. I was running the architectural firm that Joe could no longer manage. I had bills to pay. I had an all-day lecture in the morning and several clients with close deadlines. What scared me most was the fact that Joe was alone, and I was his primary caregiver. I had given so much to take care of him. If I died, what would happen to him? Lying alone in the dimmed room, I realized the enormity of the situation.

I waited for my daughters to make the five-hour drive to my bedside and wondered: Was this the price of being a caregiver? I'd been under a lot of stress that had nothing to do with my high-pressure career, my client list, and my deadlines. Caregiving had been creeping into my life day by day, minute by minute. It had started small; he'd forgotten to make the mortgage payment. The next month, I paid it. Now, I was paying all bills. In fact, I was pretty sure he couldn't figure out the bank dashboard anymore. A month ago, he had missed a critical client lunch; now I managed his calendar, sometimes calling old friends before the date to prepare them for his cognitive changes. He couldn't find his glasses, his credit card, keys, and money. Months ago, I'd responded by organizing his things on his desk, but that no longer helped. He would put his wallet in his pocket and then take it out, stashing it someplace unpredictable. These days, even giving him his wallet was dangerous. He would buy crazy things he had no use for and give money to anyone who had a sad story. I would get angry with him for being irresponsible, but that didn't help. It would frustrate me and him both. His forgetfulness had become severe. Not only did he forget information I'd just provided, like who was coming for dinner, but he no longer remembered how to bathe, brush his teeth, or shave. He cried when I helped him into the shower, saying, "I don't know what to do." It broke my heart, and I wracked my brain for some way to help him, some sign to trigger his memory, some soothing words, but nothing helped.

My caregiving responsibilities had grown exponentially as his disease progressed, and I no longer knew who I was. I thought: This is caregiving for dementia. But today I ask: Does it need to be?

HEALTH RISKS FOR CAREGIVERS

The dementia caregiver is often the second patient. Many studies report that caregivers are at high risk for physical issues, mental health issues, and even mortality.[1] Psychological symptoms include depression, anxiety, and emotional stress,[2] and these are most common among caregivers who are the patient's spouse,[3] especially among caregivers of elderly patients.[4] Physical consequences include general fatigue, digestive and eating problems, reduced immune system activity, slower recovery from injuries, relatively high levels of blood pressure, and many sleep problems.[5] As a result, these caregivers are referred to in the literature as the "hidden victims,"[6] with an explicit directive from the World Health Organization to support them and ensure their well-being during caregiving and after their relative's death.[7]

The demanding tasks of caring for someone with dementia, which require an investment of time, money, physical exertion, and mental energy, often lead to a feeling of burden among caregivers.[8] As people segue into becoming dementia caregivers and then deepen their roles as the dementia progresses, they begin to carry new economic burdens and social difficulties as their social roles change in their families and in their communities. They may feel shame, insecurity, resentment, and social isolation as a result.[9] These changes hurt caregivers' physical and mental health in addition to their economic and social well-being. In fact, caregiving burden has a negative impact on all areas of caregivers' lives.[10] These negative impacts are most severe for caregivers who are elderly themselves,[11] and this collection of findings emphasizes the enormity of chronic caregiver stress.[12]

Facts at a Glance[13]
- Physical health declined in 11 percent of caregivers.
- Chronic health issues (e.g., heart attacks, heart disease, cancer, diabetes, and arthritis) occurred in 45 percent of caregivers.
- Caregivers endured a 23 percent increase of stress hormones and a 15 percent drop in antibody level relative to non-caregivers.
- Heart disease increased by 100 percent in women who spend more than nine hours a week caring for a spouse.
- Poor eating habits occur in 58 percent of caregivers.
- Mortality rates increase by 63 percent in caregivers between the ages of sixty-six and ninety-six.

The burden of caregiving typically falls on family, and most family caregivers are women. Most of us will be asked to do it, even if it is a short request by a neighbor to look after dad while your neighbor runs to the store. My heart attack was an enormous wake-up call for me. Caregiving meant I was always on call, without a break for weekends or holidays, and without overtime pay. My cardiologist warned that if I didn't get my stress under control, it would kill me. She told me that the chronic stress associated with caregiving is equivalent to smoking a pack of cigarettes a day. Yet, what could I do? The list below provides some answers, many of which I wish I had known before my heart attack.

EDUCATE YOURSELF

Become an educated caregiver. In the age of the internet, this seems obvious, but it remains important enough to restate. As I mentioned in the introduction, many diseases present with dementia as a symptom. Consider learning everything about the type of dementia your loved one suffers from. As the disease progresses, new caregiving skills may be necessary. If you know what symptoms lie in store for your loved one, you can prepare yourself emotionally, physically, mentally, and financially for them. Knowledge will empower you, help you communicate with doctors, and prepare for the next steps. Maybe most importantly, this knowledge will enable you to differentiate the disease from the person. Being able to see your person beneath the symptoms may bring you patience and insight when you most need them. Being able to tell the disease from the person might also help you take problematic behavior less personally.

For example, if your loved one has Parkinson's dementia, learning about the unusual symptoms associated with that disease can help you. Parkinson's patients often hallucinate. If your loved one tells you that people have moved into your basement, knowing that hallucinations are behind that belief can help you derive solutions that don't include the police. That knowledge might also help you feel less personally responsible for the fact that your person sees hurtful things.

The self-education process of the caregiver is ongoing. Caregiving will require that you understand all stages of dementia. Today you might have to learn how to manage the bank dashboard, but next month you may need to learn how to fall-proof your shower stall and take over all the bill paying.

While the benefits of education seem obvious, their association with your health may surprise you. For instance, my own research shows that home-based caregivers have identified "finding available resources" as the most important source of stress relief.[14] A 2018 study showed that providing education about dementia to caregivers improved caregiver depression and their sense of burden—and it also improved behavioral and psychological symptoms of dementia in the patients. In short, providing education to caregivers of dementia patients resulted in beneficial effects for both the patients and their caregivers.[15] Another study found that after implementing an educational program, caregivers became more competent in their caregiving, and this slowed the increase in burden associated with caring.[16] Educating yourself can reduce your burden, reduce depression, and help the person you're caring for.

Adult Day Programs

You might consider adult day programs. Adult day centers offer people with dementia the opportunity to socialize and participate in activities in a safe environment. These centers can provide a chance to join staffed activities such as music, gardening, and exercise programs.[17] Perhaps more importantly, these programs can offer respite to you, the caregiver.

Dementia caregivers spend approximately nine hours each day providing care to their person, and this can lead to the detrimental health outcomes described above. Handing care duties off to professionals, while knowing your loved one is engaged in activities, provides you with "time to breathe," potentially reducing your stress.[18] Additionally, these centers are good for people with dementia. For example, attending a day center has been shown to increase survival time for men with dementia.[19] You can reduce your burden without guilt.

Similar to adult care programs, in-home dementia care can include a wide range of services such as nursing, physical therapy, bathing, dressing, and physician care. It also includes housekeeping, companion care, and recreation. It allows the person with dementia the comfort and familiarity of their home. In-home dementia care might also include asking a neighbor to sit with your loved one while you take a walk. Don't be afraid to lean on your friends and family. By reducing caregiving burdens and safely freeing up time, these services likely provide similar benefits to the caregiver as described above. You will reduce your burden and your stress—and improve your health.

As the primary caregiver, it is within your power to create a caregiving team. Include as many people as you can—friends, neighbors, family, doctors, healthcare providers, therapists, home-care agencies, support groups, meals-on-wheels, and members of your religious community. You might make new friends, and creating your team is empowering. You don't have to do it alone. A team can provide necessary assistance, emotional support, and guidance; they will help with decision-making and respite.[20]

I created a three-ring binder with tabs for each team member's phone, email, and special notes. I put it in a prominent location on the desk in the foyer where everyone could browse and add their messages. My team loved it. I had one helper write, "Joe loves to take pictures of everything," and another added, "Be sure and add cinnamon to his oatmeal." Everyone was pleased and knew that they were part of a team—especially me.

Meals-on-Wheels and Other Meal Delivery Programs

Meals-on-wheels delivers nutritious meals to seniors. They come with a smile, a safety check, and an assessment of any worrisome change that might impact wellness needs. Qualifying seniors can receive these meals free of charge. Meals can range from basic to gourmet and can accommodate many dietary restrictions.

As communicated by people with early- and mid-stage dementia, managing mealtimes becomes tricky as the disease progresses, but the aid of meals-on-wheels allows them to retain independence longer.[21] If you can use meals-on-wheels or some similar service, I urge you to do so. Not only will you reduce your burden, but you will have an opportunity to build your team and strengthen your community.

Dementia Support Groups

Support groups offer diverse topics, services, counseling, comfort, and reassurance; they can be a good source of practical advice and even humor. You can talk to other caregivers who understand what you're going through because they're in a similar situation. COVID restrictions forced many of these groups online, which proved advantageous for caregivers who found it difficult to get away. Through my support group, I learned about GPS shoe inserts that helped me track Joe when he ventured too far from home.

Research shows that support groups provide measurable benefits. One study shows that caregivers who use support groups like them and keep attending, and peer-led self-help groups improve feelings of emotional support, social contact, and control over one's life, and thus may facilitate caregiving and reduce psychological burdens.[22] Finally, support groups improve caregivers' psychological well-being, depression, burden, and social outcomes.[23]

As you have been educating yourself on your person's disease, you have probably found groups like the Alzheimer's Foundation of America, the Parkinson's Foundation, and the Dementia Society of America. Many of these national groups have local chapters, and many of these chapters offer online and in-person support groups. Your local community center may offer support groups, as might your religious group. Reaching out to these groups will add to your team and enrich your personal community.

Dementia Caregiver Training for the Family

Because family caregiving is an integral part of the care system for people with dementia, some programs offer role-training intervention to help family caregivers assume more clinical beliefs about caregiving—to take some of the problematic behaviors associated with dementia less personally—with the hope that such training offsets some of the adverse outcomes associated with caregiving.[24] Other programs can help prepare the caregiver for situations unique to dementia care by providing deeper insight into dementia diseases, understanding changes in communication and behavior, personal care and hygiene, home safety tips, fall prevention, managing their medication, and even understanding financial and legal issues.[25] As dementia progresses, training of the family caregiver becomes critical, particularly during the early and middle stages of the disease. I learned firsthand that helping my husband with dementia take a shower and get dress required training. I couldn't do it safely until a professional showed me how.

Research shows that these programs work.[26] Family members enrolled in particular training programs have demonstrated reduced stress, less personalized responses to troubling behavior, reduced depression, and reduced burden; caregivers have become less emotionally enmeshed in beliefs about caregiving roles and responsibilities.

In this book, I've tried to provide information that you can use. However, access to classes and training is limited. Sometimes you can find pilot studies through your doctors, and I urge you to ask them. You can also use the internet to search for pilot training classes for family caregivers of people with dementia. Many of the training classes offered are for professional caregivers, but some of them are free and online. You might find those useful. I wish I had tried harder to find classes for myself, or that online versions were available when I needed them.

Your Mental Health Matters

One of the best things you can do for your person with dementia is remain physically and emotionally vital yourself, which is no easy task.

The advice above relies on established groups, tools, and resources, but in the most important moments, you need to rely on yourself, on your family, friends, and the team you've built. Caregiving often means setting your own needs aside for a while—but I'm here to tell you that you need to take care of your own needs too. You will need to be kind to yourself, to set aside the guilt associated with spending a night out when your spouse can't be with you to enjoy it. You will need to set aside the worry associated with leaving your person in the hands of another caregiver. Sometimes you need help to find that kind of strength.

Therapy and counseling can help. One of the benefits accrued through the (hard-to-find) caregiving training is the emotional strength needed to see that the problematic behavior associated with dementia should not be taken personally. Professional counseling can help achieve that state too. Additionally, therapists can help parse the emotional conflicts generated by the caregiver's needs to give care, work, and take care of herself. My therapist helped me revise my priorities to address my needs and desires. (My therapist recommended a 2011 book called *The 36-Hour Day* by Mace and Rabins,[27] and I recommend it too!)

After my heart attack, my doctor referred me to an alternative physician who taught me biofeedback. We installed an app called Wild Divine by Unyte's Interactive Meditation on my computer. The program was graphic and delightful, allowing me to instantly see the benefits of changing my breathing patterns. When I was stressed, my breath was shallow, my blood pressure rose. When I breathed deeply, my blood pressure fell. After several sessions, we saw dramatic results. With the help of this app, I was able to take deep, mindful breaths in moments of stress, knowing I was actively reducing my blood pressure and the stress on my heart. It worked, and I still use it today.

Researchers have validated the benefits of counseling in numerous studies. Counseling programs for caregivers led by professionals were shown to significantly reduce the number of nursing home admissions,[28] indicating the benefits to both the caregiver and their person. Caregivers have been shown to be more able to control distressing thoughts, thereby reducing their stress, after receiving online cognitive behavioral therapy. Psychosocial interventions reduced caregiver burden and depression and delayed nursing home admission, again showing that taking care of the caregiver helps the person they are caring for. I recall going on a retreat to regain some energy I lost while caring for my husband. My absence upset his routine, and the caregiver continually called with minor problems. My retreat was hijacked, and I was left wishing I had stayed home. Looking back, rather than forgoing the retreat, I should have provided clearer directions to the caretaker and provided alternate contacts. In the moment, I felt too guilty to ask neighbors and family to serve as those alternate contacts. I felt shame that I wasn't strong enough. Therapy helped me get past that, but not until after that moment passed. I urge you to be more proactive in asking for help than I was.

Your Physical Self Matters

Once you have built a caregiving team and found the mental strength to use it, you need to take care of your physical self. The physical benefits of exercise are widely recognized, and an abundance of epidemiological evidence exists to support an association linking exercise to physical health and overall quality of life.[29] Exercise is believed to play a role in the prevention of various medical conditions such as hypertension, diabetes, cardiovascular disease, cancer, and osteoporosis, and physical activity has been shown to reduce premature mortality. Take that friend up on the offer to sit with your person and go to the YMCA, go for that walk, or go for that swim.

I found two ways to reconnect with movement. First, Joe and I took walks with our dog. Sometimes, we didn't get far, but sitting on those benches and taking those photos were terrific times. He was relaxed and happy, which allowed me to feel relaxed and happy. The opposite was also likely true—because I was relaxed and happy, he was able to be so too. Second, I found private time with my bike early in the morning while Joe was still sleeping. Riding my bike was a great way to clear my head and start the day.

Get Your Sleep, If You Can

Sleep problems for dementia caregivers are severe.[30] I would often fall asleep immediately when I sat down to watch TV, then move to the bed and find myself wide-eyed and staring at the ceiling. I would spend dark nights wondering what I could do to improve Joe's life, if I would be able to afford his care, or if I was irritating my kids or neighbors by leaning too heavily upon them for support. Knowing that sleep deprivation was causing me physical harm only increased the stress I felt while staring at the ceiling.

By using the tools described earlier in this chapter, you will feel more in control, less stressed, physically and mentally stronger, and more proactive. Those factors in themselves may help you sleep better at night. I recommend that you try them because researchers have no answers for you. In fact, researchers have identified poor sleep patterns as endemic among caregivers and suggest that sleep quality of caregivers might be a useful target for a clinical intervention.

I have the kind of advice you might find in a support group. Keep your evenings simple; avoid technology. Blue light has recently been shown to interrupt sleep patterns more than any other kind of light,[31] so consider making your room very dark or wearing blue-filtering sunglasses to bed. Your cell phone and computer generate blue light, so consider turning them off and keeping them off.

Try leaving stressful conversations for the morning. Calming activities such as meditating, praying, reading bedtime stories, and playing soft music may be helpful. I found great sleep stories on online apps (but blacken your screen!). Consider sharing these activities with your person. I also found warm lavender baths an excellent sleep aid, and chamomile and sleepytime teas warming and calming.

CONCLUSION

As you become a caregiver for a person with dementia, your personal health is at risk. You know how when you fly, the attendants tell you to help yourself first and then your children? That is my advice to you now. Take care of yourself first. Don't wait until you have a medical emergency to find support. Use education, adult day programs, in-home professional support, support groups, training, therapy, exercise, and sleep as tools to keep your body and mind resilient. Build your caregiving team broadly and deeply so that you can lean on others to fill in for you while you take care of yourself—without guilt or remorse. And remember that science shows that taking care of yourself benefits the person you are caring for.

2

A Sense of Place

It is not drawn on any map. True places never are.

—*Herman Melville*

My grandmother Clara, ninety-six, battled vascular dementia. She reached the point where she could no longer keep house or care for herself. My grandfather, ninety-eight, determined it was time to get help. He closed their family home, and together they moved to the local retirement community. When I visited, projecting my own dismay on the situation, I expected to find him gloomy and despondent, resigned to his fate. Instead, I found my grandad proud to take me on a grand tour of his "resort-style living," as he described their new community. I further anticipated that he would walk through the facility, pointing out various areas. However, he did something unexpected. Listening to his perspective all those years ago gave me insight that I still use today when I'm designing dementia care facilities and retirement communities. In his own words, Harley shared the following:

"Since Clara took sick, we moved to our new home to get help. Let me show you around." A friendly dog linked up with us, joining the grand tour. "This is our mascot, Bingo," Harley said, patting the dog. "He has free rein of the place. We all love him, and he has so many friends."

We stopped first at the chapel. Harley didn't just open the door to show me. He walked up to the front, stood behind the pulpit, and spoke. "Clara and I like our church and have already met some nice folks here." He straightened his shirt and looked out to the nonexistent crowd. "I call myself a preacher. Everyone is a preacher."

Next, we stopped at the dining room. I saw a room full of empty chairs and tables, but Harley saw more. "This is our dining room. I think everybody enjoys visiting as much as they do eating. We have 'big feeds' for something special like holidays or Mildred's birthday, and we're all invited."

We then stopped at a large bird aviary. A wheelchair sat parked in front. I saw a woman slumped over, lethargic, but Harley saw something more. "There are beautiful birds to watch inside and out. This lady likes to watch them inside. I see her here every day. Myself, I enjoy the ones outside, but I'm luckier than many folks." He bent over and greeted the woman. "I can still get around."

We walked down the hall. "Plants are everywhere here." Harley pointed to potted plants sitting inside a sun-drenched bay window. He had left a thriving garden when he'd sold his home, and I thought he might be sad about the downgrade—I was wrong. "Clara and I like to come to this spot to enjoy the afternoon sun and watch the plants grow."

We moved on to an alcove with a game table, sofa, and a couple of easy chairs, and he said, "This is a good place to talk with friends after dinner, or sometimes we play cards. My old gang from the diner comes here every Friday morning for coffee. It is our hangout." I easily imagined the old truckers and farmers with their hats and steaming mugs.

"I saved the best for the last," he said as we walked to the elevator. "It's our level." The elevator door slid open, and he gestured grandly. "On my floor, there's a nice 'red carpet.' We always feel like we're getting the 'red carpet treatment.'" He pointed to some artwork and candlesticks. "People bring some of their own things here, and it makes it feel really homey." He reached his front porch apartment entry. "And this is our place. This is my front porch. Everyone makes theirs different. I put out a little table

so I can put some of my things here, and I don't have to bend over much to pick them up."

Entering their apartment, Harley proudly announced that this was home. *"This is a good place. Friends and family can easily visit."* We walked over to the balcony and looked at the trees and street. *"From my window, I can see people coming and going, the street, the cars, and everything."* We finally sat on the sofa I recognized from their home. I also recognized their chairs, my grandmother's curio cabinet, and the artwork her son had painted. *"All our important things are here, and it feels like our home,"* Harley told me, and I could see satisfaction on his face.

Place matters.

LESSONS FROM ASSISTED LIVING FACILITIES

I recently found this story in my old journal. At the time, I was very sad to see my grandparents transition to an assisted living facility; however, Harley had a different experience. My grandmother had become tricky to care for, and he was feeling the stress of caring for both her and their home. Moving to the retirement community was both a delight and a relief. Furthermore, Harley's perception of his new place astonished me. He articulated human connections and attachments, sharing a relationship to "place" from a first-person perspective. To him, the space was more than rooms and amenities. Harley went on to thrive in this community until he died at the age of 102.

His quotes confirm what we know through scientifically supported evidence. The human connection to place, crucial to him and Clara, is significant in all senior environments. He talked about the importance of the dining room, not only for eating but also for social exchange. Art makes a place feel like home. The front porch creates a space for personal identity and welcomes family and friends. Spiritual connections depend on access to worship and foster community. Harley also identified a biophilic connection—an urge to affiliate with other forms of life—by expressing happiness with his access to Bingo the dog, birds, plants, landscape, and views.

Place science involves environmental problem-solving and uses a framework based on the understanding that our environment significantly impacts our behavior. People form emotional attachments to places, and those positive emotions can be elicited by objects associated with the place, even when people are absent from it.[1] Harley identified elements of nature, worship space, a place to socialize, and a red carpet. These elements elicited positive emotions for him, such as feelings of comfort, safety, and well-being.

Place science in the design for health and well-being has been the core of my professional work for nearly fifty years. I have seen how design provides hope in cancer centers, brings joy to children in pediatric hospitals, and provides dignity and motivation in veteran facilities. I have witnessed the reduction, hospital-acquired infection through appropriate material specification, and a decrease in medical errors through improved lighting design. Place science suggests that healing environments for people with dementia do two things: address physical needs and engage positive emotions.[2] My personal caregiving experiences has verified and refined that relationship.

We spend more than 90 percent of our time in the built environment; therefore, place is critical to our health and well-being. Most adults have opportunities to move freely from home to school or work, do shopping errands, visit the doctor and socialize with friends, and take time for recreation. For those with dementia, their connection to the world rests almost exclusively with others who can provide mobility for them. Very few people with dementia can leave home for social or other activities. Therefore, the place they live must provide all experiences for them. That's a lot to ask of a place and a caregiver. In the remainder of this chapter, I'll share with you three critical elements that benefit both you and your person, share with you reasons for why those elements are important for your mental health and the mental health of your person, and provide some ideas of how to implement elements into your lives.

ESSENTIAL PLACES

Ray Oldenburg, a sociologist, suggests that people need access to three types of places to satisfy human requirements.[3] First, and most importantly, they require a home, which is the most personal and intimate. Second, they need a place where they feel the value of contribution such as work or learning. Third, they need a place for socializing. Once these three elements are satisfied, culture, gender, and life experience will enable the other desired elements that all people, including your person, seek. In the following section, I discuss each of these elements and how you can adapt them to accommodate your person and yourself as dementia becomes a bigger factor in your lives.

First place: The concept of home is significant to everyone, even people with dementia. Aside from providing the primary link to personal identity, home is the nest, the secure place, the safe place where people retreat when things get complicated or when it's time to rest. (See chapter 4, "The Alchemy of Home.") Your person's home will have personal imagery, artifacts, clothing, and other items that your person will recognize as their own. A candy dish will remind your person of her grandmother. A turquoise bracelet will remind another person of his father. As Harley pointed out in the opening story, displaying personal items, familiar furniture, or other iconic elements helps identify the home. Household destinations require individual personalization with familiar objects to identify mementoes as having emotional attachments with specific meaning. Many personal items and artifacts have the power to bring memories of safety and love foremost into the mind of your person.

When your person with dementia is living at home, you might think you don't need to lean on the power of items to generate feelings of safety and a connection to others, but if your person loses mobility and becomes less able to access trickier parts of the house, perhaps consider how this shrinking of their world impacts their sense of home and its associated safety. You might want to move favorite photos or memorabilia from the upstairs office to the bedroom or living room if your person can no longer access the office. If you find yourself needing to move bedrooms to avoid stairs, you can minimize confusion by bringing art and other objects specific to your person. Your knowledge of your person will benefit you greatly here. Only you will know if that trophy, that painting, or that inlayed box is actually important to your person. Keeping those objects as part of the background as your person becomes less mobile will increase their sense of security and reduce confusion.

We can also lean on the power of home to help reduce the frequency of troubling behaviors. Dementia will come to affect your person's ability to deal with simple activities, including the six basic activities of daily living: eating, bathing, personal hygiene, getting dressed, toileting, and functional mobility. Families often find bath-related activities the most challenging tasks for which to provide support. I know I did. People with dementia may not remember how to do them, have movement disorders, or have poor coordination. They may have lost interest in doing things like bathing or may not understand why something like teeth brushing or handwashing needs to be done. They may not be able to understand the instructions. Both my mother and my husband forgot how to shower, and helping them with hygiene-related tasks became one of the most stressful parts of the day.

While hiring a home caregiver might seem like an obvious solution—they've taken classes on how to bathe the elderly, for example—this seldom works. Many activities of daily living, especially activities involving hygiene, invade personal space since they require intimate contact with your person. This incursion can trigger disruptive behaviors. My husband would never allow a visiting female nurse to help him in the bathroom, and my mother wouldn't allow even me, her daughter, to see her without clothing.

Home isn't just a place; home includes a sense of safety. You, as the caregiver, can rely on your knowledge of your person to help with hygiene-related tasks. You know what makes your person feel unsafe. For my mom, any form of nakedness made her feel unsafe. For my husband, realizing he didn't remember what to do in the shower made him feel unsafe. Below, I provide advice on how to keep that sense of home intact while supporting good hygiene in your person. This is the advice I wish I'd had when I was caregiving.

First, give yourself plenty of time, and only help your person with a task you know to be difficult if you are in the right frame of mind. If you're feeling crabby or short-tempered, leave the bathing for the next day. If you try to rush your person through tasks that they find frightening, confusing, and demoralizing, you will frustrate yourself and your person. For example, because my mom had forgotten how to bathe and because she hated to be seen in any stage of undress, we reduced her frequency of bathing. On a day she had a doctor's appointment, I realized that she needed a bath before I took her, but we only had an hour. Rushing her resulted in so much unhappiness that I had to reschedule the appointment.

Second, prepare your tools ahead of time as much as possible. Fill the tub with water. Lather up the sponge. Set out the towels, clean clothes, and lotions. Load the toothbrush with toothpaste. Seeing these items readied will sometimes remind your person how to engage in the task, and more importantly, you will be able to focus on keeping your person safe and happy instead of getting that washcloth out of the drawer.

Third, verbally walk your person through the tasks. Dementia impedes the brain's ability to sequence, plan, and organize multiple-step activities. It may not be enough to say, "Now brush your teeth." Instead, it may be more effective to hand a toothpaste-ladened toothbrush to your person and say, "Now put this in your mouth and move it like this." Telling your person to wash their face may be less effective than asking them to move the washcloth over their face and behind their ears. Providing step-by-step direction for my husband allowed him to maintain independence and dignity for a while longer.

Fourth, have distractions at the ready. For instance, you can have well-known music playing in the bathroom. If your person begins to show signs of agitation, you can discuss the music. I had a photo of a dog in a bathtub, and my mom and I discussed that dog and other dogs as she bathed. It distracted her and kept her happy.

Fifth, make comfort a premium. Find the softest towels, the softest underwear, the most fragrant soaps, shampoos, and lotions. If towel warmers are in your budget, consider them. With my mother-in-law, I found that I could make bath time fun by telling her it was a spa day, and I tried to include as many spa elements as a I could, placing candles on the counters, using her favorite scent, and ensuring that her robe smelled like her favorite lotion. Your person will be less unhappy about washing and dressing if they don't have to be cold, itchy, or otherwise uncomfortable. Everyone, including people with dementia, works better when relaxed and happy and surrounded by things they like.

Sixth, repetition is helpful. Establish a regular routine for the day, doing the same things at the same time. If you can, try to make sure that the problematic activity occurs at the same time. If you usually bathe in the morning, keep it in the morning. Moving it may confuse your person.

Seventh, the built environment matters. Smaller spaces are more comfortable than large open spaces for people with dementia. Covered windows are experienced as safer. Furniture design and layout can organize clothing and the dressing process for easier choices. (See chapter 5, "Furnishings Matter.") These enhancements can improve the person's emotional state and ability to understand and cooperate better.

Last, try to avoid setting yourself up for failure. Only you will know what this looks like for your person. For example, because my mom hated to be seen without clothing, I couldn't convince her to relax her standards. It didn't matter to her when I reminded her that I was her daughter, that I was a woman, that I loved her regardless of what she looked like. She would have none of it. The only way to address this issue was to accommodate it. I held up towels and used dressing screens. I filled the tub with bubbles so that once she got in, I couldn't see her. I averted my eyes when nakedness could not be avoided. Trying to ignore her worldview only ended in tears and screaming.

Home includes artifacts, but it also includes people. As discussed in chapter 1, you can lean on family members to support your person, and creating new traditions can help. A success story from a neighborhood in Iowa helps me make the case and may inspire you similarly.

Dad started to forget how to prepare his meals and found his medication too complex, so he moved in with his son and young family of football fans. The family celebrated Monday night football in the fall, and dad joined in preparing snacks and setting them out as made sense as his disease progressed. This activity included all home-based activities: food preparation, lively company, and television. He interacted alongside with his son and grandkids while the game was played, yelling at the ref with his kids. His dementia inevitably progressed, and he moved into a memory care facility. His son did not want to let the tradition go, and the Monday night football event followed dad. The facility kept those home elements intact and created a place for the event in the open atrium, bringing in iconic elements from the community, including the back end of a classic pickup truck. Tailgate picnic-style foods were provided each Monday night, and other families participated in the supper and televised ball game. This event became very so popular with the families and residents that eventually even the surrounding community participated.

What started off small and just for dad, grew to include other generations, other families, and new elements. The son in that family had patience and had the courage to invite new people, and he had the wisdom to lean on the safety and familiarity of home to make it work.

Home-based social enrichment can extend beyond special events. Kitchens encourage participation in activities like cooking and baking, putting away dishes, and sorting cutlery, and a place for storytelling, value, and connectedness. The connection can be achieved through intergenerational events, children visits, game nights, neighbors that drop by with coffee, backyard barbeques, and other social activities that bring people together to socialize. Local charities can sponsor activities, live streaming concerts, and video linking. Spiritual connectedness also provides value and empowerment.

In summary, when you lean on the power of home—the first place—
to support your person, you can lean on the memories associated with
particular items. Try to keep those items in your person's environment
as their world shrinks and changes. You can also lean on the safety and
dignity associated with home while engaged in daily tasks like bathing and eating. Be patient with yourself and don't be afraid to put off
activities for a day if you don't have the mental space to support your
person through a task likely to be tough. A bath can't wait until next
week, but it can definitely wait until tomorrow. Be patient as you try to
lean on the strong elements of home to build new traditions in support
of your person.

Second place: Work provides a feeling of value and worth. People with
dementia have generally retired from the workplace, but the motivation to contribute to the household and to society via work remains
because it fulfills the higher-level needs of esteem and self-actualization.
For people with dementia, the need for value and importance remains
strong, and there are ways for you, the caregiver, to keep that door
slightly open for your person.

Your person with dementia may have decreased abilities in both the
mental and physical arenas, but allowing your person to engage in any
kind of work can improve their mental well-being, and yours. An innovative program called Side by Side was initiated to assess the feasibility of supported workplace engagement for people with younger onset
dementia.[4] Seven people with mild dementia worked one day per week
in a large metropolitan hardware store. Work-buddies, store employees
who had undergone dementia training, worked side by side with the
person with dementia. Work duties, negotiated at the start of each shift,
included restocking, plant care, assembling display stock, and serving
customers. All participants were able to adapt to the workplace environment and some talked about "their customers." Family caregivers
reported a positive impact on self-esteem and life satisfaction as a result
of the workplace experience. This evaluation of feasibility exceeded all

expectations and demonstrated that it is possible to offer meaningful activities for people with mild dementia if an appropriate framework of support is provided.

In another example, I recall a father and son who ran a popular family restaurant we frequented. The father started to decline with dementia, but the son kept bringing his dad into the restaurant. Dad folded napkins and stacked menus. Dad felt productive and needed, and son felt like his dad was in a good place.

A similar situation occurred in my favorite clothing store. The owner had exciting fashions and a significant following of loyal customers. Her daughters continued in their mom's footsteps and managed the store with her favorite lines. When mom developed dementia, the daughters continued to bring her to the store. She spent her days chatting with her devoted clients. It worked well for them, and mom remained happy and valued until her passing.

If you do not have a restaurant or clothing store to which to take your person, consider other opportunities. For years, my father-in-law helped dry dishes after a family meal. Even in mid-stage Alzheimer's, when he rarely spoke, I found him standing at my sink looking forlorn and helpless. One night, remembering his task in the past, I handed him a dish towel while I was cleaning up. This made him break into a huge smile, and he started drying the dishes. It became a regular routine. I wish I had thought to bring my mom to her church with a rag and a can of Pledge. We would have enjoyed the time together, and the pews would still be shining. She also would have found a feeling of self-worth while volunteering in a soup kitchen, and I would have too. If your person still has the ability, and you have the time and inclination, consider volunteering at the local animal shelter, food pantry, school, or place of worship with them.

Recent research by Paul Rodgers has aimed to develop disruptive design interventions (e.g., products, systems, services, strategies) for breaking the cycle of established opinions that tend to remain unchallenged in the health and social care of people living with dementia in the

United Kingdom.[5] The long-term goal of his research was to uphold UN Article 23 that states that people have a human right to work, or engage in productive employment, and may not be prevented from doing so. Through the co-design and development of a range of products, strategies, and tools, his research provided people living with dementia who were supported by their formal and informal caregivers with innovative and creative work opportunities that shifted widely held opinions of dementia by showing that people living with dementia are capable of designing and making desirable products and of offering much to society after diagnosis. Essentially, for his research project, he involved many people with dementia and their caregivers in dementia-safe workshops where participants created innovative co-designed projects, such as football reminiscence, disruptive design workshops, exhibitions, and "pop-up" shops. These projects work for people living with dementia, addressing issues around inclusion, participation, and creativity, and giving an increased sense of self identity through activities that are carefully designed, developed, and facilitated in dementia-friendly settings. I include his research in this book to help convince you that your person may have reduced abilities, but they can still contribute, and finding a way to harness that desire may improve their mental health.

Workspaces do not need to be outside the home. Consider adapting places in your home to facilitate work. How this adaptation looks will depend on your person, but it might include a place to explore artwork or crafts, fold laundry, listen to a lecture, or empty the dishwasher. Any way that you can find to facilitate your person's ability to contribute will help them and you.

Third place: Third places are defined as spaces where people socialize, gather, and set aside activities of daily living from work or home. They exist simply for pleasure, providing a place to hang out with friendly people in a lively environment. These places are the heart of a community's social energy. According to Ray Oldenburg,[6] people require a neutral location, aside from home and work, to feel satisfied and content.

Why does your person need a third place? People, even people with dementia, feel lonely when homebound. Loneliness is defined as the perception that one's social and emotional relationships are not as strong as desired. Being homebound is significantly linked with depression, increased cognitive impairments, disruptive behaviors, and functional limitations.[7] Loneliness increases the risk of death, which is as great as smoking and obesity. Loneliness increases blood pressure and heart disease by 23 percent and increases the risk of stroke by 32 percent. Loneness advances cognitive decline.[8]

According to AARP, 90 percent of seniors over the age of sixty-five want to remain in their own home. Many people find the prospect of moving into a care facility terrifying, and research suggests people don't fear losing their house as much as they fear losing their community, their friends, neighbors, grocery stores, place of worship, their bank, and their mail delivery person. They fear losing their entire world as they know it. Aging in place, moving in with family, or moving to a care facility is a dramatic experience because people fear losing their social networks.

Nearly one-third to one-half of our seniors feel lonely or experience social isolation. People with dementia have a higher risk of becoming socially isolated and lonely because their ability to access the outside world depends on you, their person. Losing the ability to drive or access public transportation can increases loneliness. Physical frailty and cognitive impairment can impede the ability to maintain connections with our friend networks.[9] Reducing loneliness in your person is a big ask, but the remainder of this chapter offers some advice.

Keeping your person with dementia active and engaged in the community promotes mental health—and the third place can help. Our understanding of what drives health and happiness tells us that obesity shortens our lives, while antibiotics, physical activity, and healthy diets prolong it. New findings tell us that our relationships with the people we know and care about are just as critical to our survival.[10] Face-to-face contact can make us healthier and happier.

Let's take a closer look at the third place. Like home and work, what the third place looks like for your person will depend a lot on your person. Third places might include parks, breweries, coffee shops, pubs, shopping malls, fast-food establishments, and many other places. Oldenburg[11] argues that the third place is vital for civil society, democracy, engagement, and, most importantly, establishing a sense of place. The third place can mitigate social isolation for your person with dementia.

The importance of the third place was recently made clear to me. When I was working on a recent Veteran Affairs project, a vet voiced his request for a "Times Square." After I asked him to describe it, I realized that he and his friends wanted a place to hang out. What he was wanted was a third place. Taking the lead from his age and his descriptions of the perfect Times Square, my team and I designed a gathering place with a clock tower and casual seating between three households. The space included a dog mascot to hang out with them.

Looking back, I see that my grandfather was able to continue his relationship with his fantastic third place late into his nineties. When his buddies could no longer drive, but he was still able, Harley would gather them up and drive them to the local diner. There, they would tell stories about the farm days, the wars, and the state of the Union. The local diner provided great value in their lives by keeping relationships intact. Furthermore, he was able to move his third place into the retirement community.

When seeking a third place for you and your person, you might start by considering the obvious places. Because so many retailers have seen value in providing a cherished third place (watch any Starbucks commercial), many potential third places are accessible to those with reduced mobility, and this supports healthy aging. Paneras and Whataburgers actively solicit people to hang out in their spaces.

If your person already has a third place, see if you can keep taking them there, even as the dementia progresses. Old friends are kind friends, and they will support your person while you take care of yourself. If you are at a loss when it comes to finding a third place, don't be afraid to ask the support team you built in chapter 1. Ask your local dementia support groups and people at your place of worship. Adult day care centers can also support this need.

When looking for the right place, Oldenburg recommends that third-place spaces should include the following:

1. Accessibility: The third place is visible, easy to find, and accessible to the elderly with disabilities, walkers, wheelchairs, canes, and scooters. Furniture should be easy to get around and flexible, where the patrons can customize seating arrangements. Typically, third places have extended hours and are available throughout the day and evening, allowing people and their buddies to come at their preferred time.
2. Welcoming: The friendly atmosphere should be apparent to all visitors. The place should welcome grandchildren, out-of-town visitors, and those who are new. There should be iconic images or descriptors so that all will recognize as the space as a third-place destination.
3. Comfortable atmosphere: Rooms and alcoves should provide cozy and comfortable areas that support informality and casualness. Adjacent gardens, outdoor spaces, fireplaces, and books can help create a relaxing atmosphere.
4. Familiar faces: Third-place spaces are places to see and be seen. Temporary encounters of friendships can provide new bases for authentically relating. Through dignity and authenticity, friendship can contribute to mental health and reduce loneliness.[12] Meeting up with friends, even for your person with dementia, can reduce loneliness.
5. Facilitated interactions: When looking for the optimum third place, consider seeking the following elements or adding them yourself. Windows can provide a focal point to encourage dialogue on the weather and the sight. Newspapers can provoke discussion on the day's headlines. Other props, such as seasonal décor items, photos, and vintage artwork, can be helpful conversation starters.
6. Refreshments: Light refreshments can provide an attraction, social stimulant, and support for the comfort factor. While meals are unnecessary, coffee and beverages, light snacks, and cookies are great socializers.
7. Neutral location: Third places exist on neutral ground and provide social equality and inclusion.

Ultimately, third places support healthy aging for you and your person with dementia by providing opportunities for meaningful engagement, sociability, and contributing roles.[13]

Traveling with Your Person

Those with dementia may not articulate the desire to travel, but they retain the ability to engage in the experience.[14] You may wonder if you can travel with your person, and I can speak from firsthand experience that you can. It can be therapeutic for both of you, especially if you manage your expectations beforehand.

Jan Dougherty wrote a great book on this topic called *Travel Well with Dementia: Essential Tips to Enjoy the Journey*.[15] She offers calm and familiarity as guiding principles. For example, when booking accommodations, seek room configurations that look like those at home, and place personal items in similar locations. Close the curtains at night so that shadows are not mistaken for strangers in the room, and take measures to prevent your person from leaving the room and wandering off. I suggest that during longer bouts of travel, bring out magazines, puzzles, or movies on tablets to occupy your person. Snacks may distract your person and help avoid sudden confusion, frustration, and arguments. I suggest private, shorter excursions work better than larger group excursions, and dining arrangements with four or fewer settings also work better. This principle also applies to visiting or hosting family and friends, where separate lodgings nearby facilitate quiet time and uninterrupted rest periods. Another tip is to take a daily photo of your person in their travel clothes in case they get lost and you need to identify them.

As a seasoned traveler, I traveled with Joe to a resort in Mexico in his middle stages of dementia. It was our last trip together, which I will remember with great fondness. He laughed, enjoyed the varied restaurants, the beach, and Mariachi entertainers, and together we had a great time. However, it was not without challenges. There were times when he needed a great deal of reassurance, and I found that things went more smoothly when I worked with his comfort level. For instance, when he decided he was finished with his meal—even before the main course was served—we left. When he became angry about the art in our suite—"Why did we ever pick such awful art?"—I had what I hoped was a reassuring smile, held his hand, and suggested that we get a snack. Arguments or trying to explain the reality would not help in any circumstance. The trip was worth the difficulties, and the good times outweighed the challenges. I'm so glad we made that trip.

Restaurants provide another kind of travel, and they can help keep community ties intact for your person. Dining with your loved one can be difficult for the caregiver; however, a little planning can greatly improve the experience for all. Consider selecting a restaurant that is familiar and that has quick service. Perhaps plan to arrive before or after the main rush. You might call ahead and explain your needs and seating preferences. Ask the host for a seating area that is quiet and without traffic and distractions. Window views are helpful during the day. Choose a seating area that is secluded, with corners, alcoves, booths, or outdoors.

Once you're there, engage them in conversation. Conversations that include memories from when your person was young have a higher likelihood of success. I also found that bringing along treats—my person's cell phone and a camera loaded with old photos—could distract my person while waiting. Because the attention span in people with dementia is limited, agitation may develop. The saltshaker may end up in the water glass and sugar packets in the soup—do not fret. People are kind, and if you call ahead, servers understand. You can get "to-go boxes" and move to a picnic at home.

CONCLUSION

Even though your person has dementia, and you may feel your world shrinking as their does, you have ways to keep your world big. You can lean on elements of home to ameliorate troubling behavior and to ease transitions into new spaces. You can lean on elements of work life and help your person keep some self-esteem by seeking out tasks and engaging your person with them. And you can lean on elements of community, keeping social ties intact for as long as possible. Travel will be different, but it remains possible; if you're considering it, I recommend Jan Dougherty's 2019 book. And as always, be kind and patient with yourself. You cannot care for your person if you can't care for yourself.

3

Trigger Factors

The ER doctor looked at me, "I can see you have problems with him."

He wasn't wrong. I'd gone to the restroom, leaving Joe alone in the exam room for fewer than five minutes. As I walked back, my stomach churned. Paper cups and crumpled paper lay on the floor outside the room. Clearly, he had thrown them. Magazines, brochures, and even the rack that held them were scattered in the room and in the hall outside the room. His shoes and socks? Joe had thrown them all out the door.

It had happened before. Joe threw stones over the fence at a slightly annoying neighbor. He threw napkins across the table and even a cup of coffee at a retirement party. He didn't appear to be aiming—only throwing. Why?

It had been a long day in the Emergency Department, and we were both tired and ready to go home. I was too exhausted to confront Joe. When I finally entered the exam room, I found my husband devastated and exhausted, but his eyes lit when I touched him.

"I'm so happy to see you! I didn't know where I was, and I couldn't get anyone to come," he said.

Too tired for scolding or questions, I gave him a hug and helped him with his shoes and socks.

I understood the trigger then. Joe had tried to communicate with the hospital staff, trying to communicate with actions when he didn't have words. I suddenly understood his other outbursts too. When he threw things, he was struggling to connect.

Discovering this trigger allowed me to reduce future throwing events. When I saw Joe becoming frustrated in a conversation, I handed him his camera—he would never throw his prized possession. When that was not on hand, I gently took his arm and suggested a walk, removing him from a tense situation. I was fortunate to identify the trigger for Joe's behavior. It isn't always possible.

SUPPORTING YOUR PERSON WITH DEMENTIA

I wish that, in this section, I could tell you how to magically identify the trigger that sets off your person—the thing that inspires the disruptive behavior—but the fact is, we often don't know. I wish I could tell you how to magically calm your person each time they get triggered, but that can be challenging too. However, I can offer some pathways to hope, some ways that can help you and your person. Some of these pathways come from publications written by professional caregivers. Others come from my own experiences and from interviews with family caregivers. I wish I'd known most of them when I was caring for my people.

You, as the family caregiver, have a significant advantage in successfully implementing interventions—because you already know your person. You appreciate their background culture, where they have been in their life, understand likes and dislikes, and know emotional hot buttons. You, and other family caregivers, can translate body language and other nonverbal clues. You, and your team, have likely already created interventions based on personal connections.

By engaging emotions in a purposeful way, environmental space has the potential to support healing. In her book *Healing Spaces*,[1] Esther Sternberg describes how the senses play a crucial role in defining the world's perception. "With the modern techniques of biochemistry, cell biology, and molecular biology, we can piece together how the elements of the world react around us, which we perceive through our sense. These perceptions trigger different brain areas, generating feelings of awe, fear, peace, and comfort. These emotions, when blended, can promote healing."

As described in chapter 1, by improving the lives of people with dementia, you also improve the physical and mental health of yourself, the family caregiver, and this improves the life of your person with dementia. "Disruptive behavior" is such a simple tag for behaviors that can be gut wrenching. No one wants to watch their person bang their head on the wall or listen to their person tell police that rapists are living in their basement. Regardless of what we call this, these dementia-based behaviors can pull loved ones down the rabbit hole, creating high-stress situations. In chapter 1, I have provided tips on how to protect yourself. In this chapter, I provide recommendations to interrupt or prevent disruptive behaviors. The changes I can recommend are generally simple, inexpensive, and practical.

The Problem: Disruptive Behavior

This chapter opens with a vignette showing disruptive behavior. Anyone who has cared for someone with dementia has been collateral damage by such a disruption. The outburst can make the caregiver feel helpless and alone. It can raise your blood pressure and generate stress. It can disrupt other people, especially if the person with dementia lives in a care facility or with extended family. No one wants their grandkids to watch granddad bang his head on the wall. Disruptive behaviors by people with dementia are among the most difficult challenges of caring for people with this syndrome.

Behavior—disruptive or otherwise—is a form of communication, and communication is adaptive for all people, generally helping us to fulfill particular needs. When language and reason are limited, communication is likely to be overtly behavioral. As people with dementia progress to lose their language and reason, behavior will increasingly become the primary method of communication. Even when speech is

intact, verbal communication is often limited by difficulties in expressing thoughts correctly. Cognitive impairment and loss of appropriate
filters disturb verbal skills, thus triggering disruptive behavior. People
with dementia often struggle to communicate feelings and needs.

Protecting Yourself by Managing Expectations

I want to use this section to offer some advice on what not to do,
and why going into the dark places I'm going to describe is unhelpful
to both you and your person. For starters, labeling behaviors as "bad"
or "unwanted" negates the adaptation that might be inherent in the
behavior. When a baby cries because she's hungry, we don't label that
behavior as disruptive—the baby needs to cry so that we know it's time
to feed her—and yet the baby and your person have similar language
abilities. I know the professionals use "disruptive," but maybe you can
find a better word to use in your own house and with your own team.
Negative labels can foster a sense of futility in both your person with
dementia and yourself.

Here is one thing I wish I'd known while I was caregiving: people
with dementia typically lack the cognitive skills to manipulate you with
their behavior. Instead, behavioral issues arise from the disease process
and the resulting coping and communication styles that often resemble
those more commonly seen in young children. It's important to remember this when you feel fed up with your person.

I remember one time when Joe was in his early stages of dementia.
We had scheduled an important client phone call. I reminded him just
before the call started. I'd provided him with a magazine and something
to drink, and yet he rudely interrupted the call, shouting a demand for
a second drink while I was negotiating tricky schedules on the phone.
I was overwhelmed with the certainty that Joe was purposefully derail-
ing the meeting because he was trying to undermine me. I was so angry
that I threw my glasses at him. In retrospect, I understand that he didn't
have the ability to purposefully undermine me, much less the desire.
His disease had simply found an unfortunate time to intrude into my

life. My hope for you is that when your person's disease intrudes into your life, you can remember that your person doesn't have the ability to manipulate. And if you don't remember, and you throw your glasses, I hope you are kind to yourself and move quickly past the moment. I also hope you realize that people with memory and reasoning problems aren't going to feel remorse for something they said or did because they don't remember that they said or did it, and they wouldn't understand the implications even if they did remember.

By definition, people with dementia have an impaired ability to learn or reason. Try to avoid the trap that comes from thinking that you can teach your person new information or reorient them to adapt to their skill loss. You'll likely end up frustrating both yourself and your person. When my mom developed Parkinson's-based dementia, one of the first skills she lost was her ability to read a calendar. I remember searching stores for an easier calendar, which of course doesn't exist. I remember trying to walk her through the days of the week, pointing to the calendar on the wall. It didn't end well because the calendar wasn't the problem, and she wasn't going to relearn the skill.

If you remember that your person isn't manipulating you, that your person cannot apologize, and that you can't reteach or reorient your person, you will be many steps ahead of where I was. You will be kinder to yourself, and this will enable you to be kinder to your person.

The Cause: Triggers

Disruptive behavior may seem to come out of nowhere, but in one study, a triggering factor was observed in 57 percent of this behavior.[2] While symptomatic of dementia, these behaviors typically result from feeling scared, paranoid, angry, confused, pained, or frustrated with an inability to communicate needs.[3] Under-stimulation and overstimulation can also lead to unwanted behavior. Consider how you would feel in the following scenario: You start your day feeling irritable, angered, or depressed, then remove the tools you might use to handle these situations, including reason, speaking skills, and understanding. You want to experience a newspaper, a cup of tea, the reduction of television noise, you are hungry—but you can't tell anyone. Unable to communicate, you too might disrupt the space. Looking back, I'm sure Joe interrupted my telephone meeting because he was bored.

Triggers may result from multiple sources and interacting factors; they typically fall into three categories: medical, psychological, and environmental. Medical triggers can result from pharmaceutical side effects and physical pain that your person can't describe. For example, the onset of an influenza infection causes inflammation, which causes depression.[4] Your person can't tell you that their stomach hurts. The stomach pain could trigger a disruptive behavior. This book doesn't directly address medical triggers, but caregivers should be aware that medical issues could be the sources of stimuli.

Psychological triggers can occur via communication. Asking someone with dementia a question for which they lack words to answer, or for which they don't know the answer, can generate anger. For example, someone may ask, "Does your daughter live nearby?" The person with dementia might not remember where their daughter lives. This question may cause anxiety and elicit disruptive behavior. The person with dementia may not remember their daughter or start a search for the missing daughter. The person with dementia may start crying, thinking harm has come to their daughter. Asking questions of a person with dementia rarely provides useful information and often leads to additional stress. Eliminating questions was one of the most challenging issues for me to understand. Questions can seem so benign and helpful, but for a person with dementia, questions can be highly stressful.

Environmental triggers pertain to elements within the place, such as lighting, windows, furniture, colors, and sounds. For example, suppose the person with dementia cannot decode the cues indicating where the bedroom or bathroom can be found. Clothing and noise can be triggers; for example, uncomfortable clothing or loud noise can overstimulate them, and they may respond with disruptive behavior. Multiple elements within the environment may be irritating. Yet, the person with dementia may not be able to communicate that it is too cold or that the beeping noise is driving them crazy.

Interventions

In this section, I offer potential interventions. Some of these might help you interrupt behavior—and connect with your person—before unwanted behavior occurs. Sometimes, you will fail. Please be kind to yourself if and when this happens. Even if you can reduce the frequency of unwanted behavior, you yourself will be calmer and happier.

The use of intimate knowledge: You, as a home-based caregiver, are likely already proficient at preventing and ameliorating disruptive behavior with the use of positive triggers.[5] For example, one woman caregiver who cared for her husband at home said,

> *My husband got very agitated when I began to make dinner. He started going through the trash, spilling the contents everywhere. I tried to stop the problem by emptying the trash before I cooked dinner, but that didn't help. He responded by pulling things out of the drawers and closet. Finally, I remembered how he enjoyed reading the paper before dinner. I gave him newspapers while I cooked, and we were both happy.*

She was able to draw on a lifetime of memories in conjunction with the pattern of his disruptive behavior to deduce what her husband wanted, even though he didn't have the words to communicate them. Remember that, when you're trying to make sense of your person's vexing behavior, studies can find triggers in only 57 percent of the cases. If you can't find a solution, like handing your person a newspaper, be kind to yourself. You might just have to ride it out.

The use of common cultural knowledge: Confusion in a person with dementia can occur from misreading environmental cues that people without dementia take for granted, such as coming home and checking the mail. A person with dementia may recall the routine and refuse to go through a door, needing to check the mail—only to find no mailbox where they expect one to be. They cannot communicate the need to check the mail or the expectation of a letter from their son. They may use disruptive behavior, saying this isn't their home and refusing to enter. Solutions can be as simple as entering through a different door or walking away from the door and returning, explaining, "Now we're going home. I have your key, and I am unlocking your front door, and we can go inside and read the mail." Keeping to a prescribed routine with supportive iconic elements helps reduce triggers.[6]

As your person's disease progresses, providing clues to support the function of a room might be helpful. For example, a person with dementia may stand in the center of a bathroom without understanding what they are supposed to do. They may become stressed when they are disrobed. Telling the person, "It's time to take a bath," is rarely helpful. Adding pictures on the wall of bathing scenes, a basket of towels, and bath objects like a bath brush, sponge, or bathrobe may provide necessary clues that allow the person with dementia to decode the expectations. It can help the caregiver communicate that bath time is imminent.

Easy environmental changes: Reflective surfaces such as mirrors, windows, and glass doors, which might present distressing or unrecognizable images, provide common triggers.[7] Try using mirrors only over sinks or in grooming areas that often make sense to those with dementia; avoid mirrors that can be seen from a distance or while walking, which can present images that are harder to understand. The same is also true for windows.

My own mom saw neighborhood lights reflected in her dining room window, and she became certain that some experimental lab was being set up and that they only operated at night. Closing the drapery before dark solved the problem. Drapery or window coverings can conceal the glass at night, which may cast distracting images.

Reflections on floors can also cause stress. Border floor patterns can be confused with steps. The reflection of lights in flooring can be misread as objects to avoid. Reflections of light with moveable objects, such as ceiling fans, cast moving shadows that can be distressful and frightening. Be mindful of all items that create shadows, reflections, or movement.

Strange noises surround us in our everyday world. Our microwaves, the doors on our refrigerators, the timers on our washing machines and dryers, our computers, and our robotic vacuums continually remind us of their presence and function with beeps and buzzes, and sometimes recorded voices. Those with dementia rarely understand them.[8] One woman in my study confused the sound of her refrigerator door being left open with her home doorbell.[9] Consider going on a mindful noise hunt to track down and eliminate these annoying sounds.

Because communication has evolved to help us meet needs, and because behavior is a kind of communication, when your person uses disruptive behavior to communicate, don't forget the basics. If your baby was crying, you might ask yourself if the infant is too warm, too cold, too hungry, or too thirsty. If your person is using disruptive behavior, consider starting with the same basics. You can then move on to stomach aches, itchy clothes, and other less obvious discomforts.

Social interventions: Despite progressive cognitive loss, people with dementia retain basic human needs, including the need to belong, the need to be loved, the need to be touched, and the need to feel useful.[10] The team you built in chapter 1 can help make up for the deficit caused by the fact that appropriate social groups are often unavailable. They can hang out with your person, touch their shoulder, and talk about old times, especially if you prompt them to avoid questions.

You as the caregiver can also help bolster feelings of usefulness by giving them chores based on their interests and abilities. Folding laundry, sorting socks, sorting flatware, and filling pots with soil can keep hands and minds busy while fostering feelings of usefulness. Planned activities should be "failure free," promoting a sense of success by accommodating the ability level of your person.[11] Even if they pair orange socks with blue, remember that retraining and reorienting are futile tasks. Any activity that engages hands and minds is a success, regardless of the outcome.

Researchers warn us of a pitfall that we can avoid by using social interventions. By reinforcing problematic behavior with attention and ignoring independent behavior, caregivers might be fostering disability or aggressive behavior.[12] A person with mild dementia who can still dress themselves and brush their teeth might be agitated by a caregiver who wants to do it for them. By engaging people with dementia with common tasks, we can ensure that they do not lose abilities prematurely.

Redirection: We can redirect people engaged in unwanted behavior to a more desired behavior, thereby using one of the most used tools in professional dementia care.[13] However, researchers have found that redirection can often generate aggressive behavior in the person with dementia, probably because the person with dementia is using the behavior to try to communicate. Your person might be unable to communicate their goal, or their goal might be nonsensical, but they are likely using their behavior to achieve a goal. This means that redirection is not as straightforward as you might have hoped when you started reading this section.

Redirection might be best approached as a multistep process. Researchers suggest that caregivers start by validating the emotions of the agitated person. You might start with something like, "You look worried," or "You seem upset." This builds rapport in the moment with your person. Next, you, the caregiver, should engage in the behavior with your person. "You look like you're looking for the kids. I'm looking for something too. Maybe we could look together." Once you have a common goal, you can engage in a distraction. "We could look in the park. Let's walk there." If your person has attention problems or difficulty with short-term memory, distraction is very effective and easy to implement. Finally, you can use your redirection. "This sure is a lovely park. I'm glad we're here." According to researchers, this multistep process saves times because you don't need to manage overly disruptive behavior.[14] I myself didn't know about this multistep approach when I was caregiving, but I know that I could have successfully implemented it many times.

Plan for a decline: Researchers describe people with dementia as having a progressively lowered stress threshold (PLST). This means that people with dementia have difficulties receiving, processing, and responding to environmental stimuli due to the progressive deterioration in cognitive, affective, and functional abilities that accompanies dementia.[15] PLST means that stimuli that barely register with the senses of an unimpaired person can trigger disruptive behavior in a person with dementia. The PLST model, introduced into dementia care in 1981, was designed to teach care providers to organize observations to make care decisions and plan care by modifying stress-inducing triggers. The PLST model proposes that caregivers modify the environmental conditions of people with dementia as they experience progressive cognitive decline so that cues can be more easily processed and are, thus, less stressful. For you, this means that as dementia progresses, you might need to adjust your approach to the decline.

Care principles may be a helpful guide in dealing with disruptive behaviors. Six principles of care are practical to assist caregivers in managing levels of stress as dementia progresses: (1) maximize safety around the home as motor functions deteriorate as dementia progresses; (2) provide unconditional positive reinforcement; (3) gauge anxiety, avoidance, and stimulation levels before engagement or activities; (4) observe and listen to those with dementia, listen and observe their body language; (5) modify environments to support losses and enhance safety; and (6) engage in ongoing education, participate in support groups, and share caregiving tips and problem-solving ideas with other caregivers. While these precepts were developed for professional caregivers, they can work for you too.

Wandering and Its Triggers

Wandering, defined as moving from place to place without a fixed plan, sounds harmless, but this behavior frequently includes accidents, getting lost, rummaging through others' personal belongings, and elopement.[16] People with dementia wander while dressed inappropriately for the weather, and they wander into traffic and can become lost and unable to find their way back home. Six out of ten people with dementia will wander. When people with dementia wander, they sometimes forget how to get to a specific place or where they are. As a result, they become lost, confused, frustrated, and often frightened. Wanderers have three times the fall rate as non-wanderers. Because of the danger associated with this behavior, it is frequently managed with physical restraints or medications,[17] which is stressful for people for all.

Wandering presents in different forms, often with other triggers. The following intervention suggestions may help mitigate wandering.

- **The problem: wandering:** Agitated pacing and restlessness are often triggered by the inability to do something or not wishing to do something, such as taking a bath.[18]
- **Intervention:** Engage the person with dementia in a task. Ask them to help set the table, sort the socks, or help stack the books. Positive distractions help relieve restlessness.
- **The problem: sundowning:** Consistent wandering in the hours of sunset.[19]
- **Intervention:** Consider exposure to morning light to reset the circadian clock. Preventing people with dementia from experiencing the changes in light associated with late afternoon and early evening reduced a series of disruptive behaviors. Chapter 4, "The Joy of Nature," describes how to work with the internal biological clock.
- **The problem: nighttime wandering:** Consistent wandering at nighttime, while asleep, is often considered a sleep problem.[20]
- **Intervention:** Mitigation for night wandering is typically pharmaceutical; however, bright light therapy upon awakening has been considered helpful to reset the body clock. Bright light therapy is

used to manage circadian rhythm disorders such as sleep problems. The therapy exposes the individual to morning light upon awakening to gradually shift sleep patterns. See chapter 6: "Light for Dementia."

- **The problem: elopement:** Leaving one's home, no longer recognizing home as the place they live, or trying to find another location or person are not only some of the most distressing dementia symptoms, but they can also lead to accidents, anxiety, and even death. Elopement is one of the most severe characteristics of wandering.[21]
- **Intervention:** Dementia-based technology such as door alarms, ankle or wrist bracelets, and GPS shoe inserts can be helpful. See chapter 8, "Technology for Dementia."

Like other disruptive behavior, wandering has its triggers. Wandering behavior can be interpreted as the person with dementia saying, "I feel lost," "I'm searching for something I've lost," or "I'm looking for someone or some place." While mitigating wandering behavior in people with dementia is particularly challenging, consider a four-step human-centric approach:

1. Identify the individual patterns of your person; study the path they wander on. Where are they going and when are they going there?
2. Try to identify the trigger that may have led to episodes, such as agitation, medication, interaction with another person, or an environmental barrier. Try to eliminate the triggers.
3. Engage in a positive distraction or use an appropriate design intervention. For example, ask your person to fold socks or sort the laundry when they start demonstrating the agitation that foreshadows wandering. Use light therapy to prevent the initial agitation.
4. Reassure your person and promote the person's dignity, freedom, and safety.

Example from a memory care facility: Environmental design interventions can address wandering in creative ways adapted by the family caregiver. Memory Care Village in Cedar Rapids and Marion, Iowa, and Greeley, Colorado, designed a safe-wandering program to allow residents to wander through loops of specially designed experiential spaces that were familiar, interesting, safe, and enjoyable. The circuit included Montessori engagement stations, familiar iconic landmarks from the community, and places to rest and socially engage. The center uses Montessori activities with popular destinations. These programmed pathways allow those with dementia to wander without fear of getting lost or harmed.

Based on these, family caregivers might consider creative ways to let their loved ones safely wander. Walking the dog and strolling the park with a companion are good alternatives for wandering. My mom loved going to her favorite shopping mall and wandering from shop to shop, often stopping to pick something up, feel the fabric, and then continue. There was always a must-stop at the pastry shop. I let her choose the destinations without a purpose. Suggesting we needed to buy a pair of shoes could often lead to frustration and confusion unless she decided she wanted to try shoes on. I had similar outings in the neighborhood with my late husband, and I found that keeping the excursions short and in very tight areas that he enjoyed in the past created the least amount of stress.

CONCLUSION

Caregiving isn't easy. If it were, we wouldn't see so many health risks associated with it. Some of the advice offered in this chapter requires a small change in your life. For example, close your drapes before it gets dark. Others will require muscle memory. For example, memorize the four steps for quick and easy redirection. Others will require some practice. Through your journey, I urge you to remember that disruptive behavior is a form of communication, and you have some power to reduce its occurrence by anticipating triggers before they start and just as they start. When you fail—and we all fail—remember that your person isn't doing this to manipulate you, and that they can't apologize for their behavior. When you fail, be kind to yourself and to your person. Consider keeping track of your successes instead of your failures.

The Alchemy of Home

There's no place like home; there's no place like home.

—*Dorothy*

After a pleasant trip together, my mom and I stood in the baggage claim area of O'Hare Airport, waiting for our bags.

"Are we home?" she asked.

"Almost. I still need to pick up the bags and the car and drive us to your house."

"But I want to go home."

She reminded me of a toddler, so I channeled that kind of patience and pulled out the tools that I would use for a small child.

"We'll get there," I said. "We have to get our bags first."

She didn't say anything. I was tired and hungry too, and the trip from the airport to her house would take about an hour, once we were in the car. I felt relief when I saw the baggage carousel moving. I felt less relief when I saw the passengers mobbing it. I didn't want to take mom into that throng.

"Mom, wait right here, and let me get the bags." I pointed to make sure she understood.

"I want to go home," she said.

"We're working on in."

I went to retrieve the bags, but when I returned, she was gone. Panicked, I dragged her bag and mine to a phone. An airport official brought her back to me, almost right away—but the damage was done.

Mom was fully agitated now. "I want to go home—where mom is." The airport official helped me get her and the bags to the car, but the ordeal was about to explode.

"Okay," I said, to calm her.

Considering her mom had died more than forty years ago, her request was impossible. I buckled her seatbelt, but she didn't want it buckled.

"We're going home," I said. "I promise."

My words meant nothing to her. Mom was convinced that I wasn't taking her home, that I didn't know where home was. She wanted to get home right now, even if she had to do it herself.

"You don't know where home is," she said in a tone she used when things were about to get rough. "You're kidnapping me."

We were driving now. I really wanted to get her home.

"Mom." I touched her arm and took my eyes off the road long enough to look at her. "It's me. Barb. Your daughter. I'm not kidnapping you."

"You don't know where home is."

"I do," I said, leaning on the same tools I had for my kids when they were little. "It's in LaPorte and we'll be there in about forty-five minutes."

"LaPorte!" She was almost shouting. "My mom isn't in LaPorte." She unbuckled herself—while I was driving fifty-five miles per hour—and started climbing over the seat. "I want to go home!"

I was scared now. I couldn't drive like this. I hit the automatic lock button and pulled into a truck stop.

"Mom!" I was shouting now too. "Stop it!"

But stopping wasn't on her agenda. The minute I pulled the car into park, she opened the door, bolted out like a rabbit, and started running between the semitrucks.

"Someone take me home!" She banged on tires and bumpers as she sprinted. "I need a ride home!"

Some kind soul saw what was happening and corralled my poor mom. I rushed over to them, relieved that she hadn't been hit by a truck, scared that I couldn't drive with her, and angry that she was behaving this way.

"I just want to go home," my mom explained to the trucker. "And she—" Mom pointed an accusing finger at me. "She doesn't know how to get there."

The trucker looked at her and then at me, easily assessing the situation. "I'm sure she does, ma'am," the trucker said.

Mom wasn't having it. "You don't know either!" She was crying now.

Finally, I called my brother, who lived in LaPorte. I explained what was happening, and he asked to talk to mom.

She recognized his voice, and when he reassured her that I knew how to find my way, she calmed a bit and got back into the car. Thankfully, the ordeal had exhausted her. She slept all the way back.

The deep-seated desire to go home plagued my mom for the rest of her life. She longed to return to her emotional home filled with love and family. Sometimes she remembered that her own mom was dead, but it didn't matter. Later, as her dementia progressed, she would sometimes refuse to go into her own house, insisting it wasn't her home. Then, in the later stages of dementia, she would escape from her assisted living residence. Once she actually climbed over a chain-link fence, and another time she escaped through a basement door, stymying the ankle bracelet they'd put on her to make sure she didn't leave. When the authorities asked her what she was doing, she always said the same thing: she wanted to go home.

What was my mom searching for? How can we help our people with dementia find it? Can we help them recognize it in their current abode?

THE EMOTIONAL HOME: WHAT IT MEANS TO WANT TO GO HOME

Home as a concept seems so simple. As children, it's the first drawing we make—a little box with the chimney on top, a window, and a front door. It has little stick figures of a smiling family in front of it. A long-rayed sun in the sky. Sometimes we add birds in the sky or pets in the grass. From the time we were children, we knew what home was.

But do we?

For people both with and without dementia, going home is a frequent wish often expressed in times of loneliness, frustration, fatigue, and anxiety. When we grow up and leave the place of our childhood, part of us stays. Our early homes continue to live in our minds and our hearts, and they morph throughout our lives, even if we don't develop dementia. Sometimes we long for our actual home. Sometimes we long for our childhood home. Maybe we long for the home in which we raised our children. The essence of home varies with individuals and time, and for those with dementia, it may vary throughout the course of the disease. The need to find home is deep and emotional, and it is always with us.[1]

Home has two aspects. First is the structural dwelling, and second is the emotional spot. Because homes have a difficult-to-describe alchemy, people often can't describe it well. How would you describe a beloved home to a friendly stranger? You might start off with physical descriptions and then end with something like, "I don't know. It was just a great house."

For people with dementia, that emotional attachment remains in place, but cognitive impairment makes it difficult for them to correctly link the emotional attachment to an existing location. Without dementia, we might simply enjoy the pleasure of nostalgia without the desire to travel to a spot. With dementia, we want to actually return to the past.

Out of love, we try to fill the lives of the people we love with things and experiences that make them happy. When our person with dementia wants to go home, we want to make that happen for them—but it's almost always an impossible request. Our person with dementia can't go to the home in their hearts and memories because the people they associate with home may have passed or grown, the physical house may have been torn down, or the house may have been updated so that it now lacks familiar landmarks.

Our person with dementia might set out on a quest for that home-based comfort and security—for a home that no longer exists—and that quest can generate behaviors that are stressful to the caregiver and dangerous to your person. A desire for home may lead to looking for home, and that often triggers wandering, elopement, and obsessive searching through cabinets or other items. A desire for home might lead your mom to run through a truck stop like a cat just let out of a bag. These are terrifying experiences for caregivers.

Even when our person is comfortable in their own home, we might hear, "I want to go home." It can be heartrending to you, the caregiver, as you try to explain that they *are* home. My mother once spent an hour crying on my adult daughter's shoulder, telling her that she wanted to go home, and when my daughter tried to tell her that she'd be going home soon, my mother launched into heartbreaking sobs and described her childhood home, a place my daughter knew no longer existed. She felt like a terrible caregiver, like she had let her beloved grandmother down. It didn't matter that the request was impossible; the sorrow didn't stop until my daughter told my mom that they'd go on a road trip to find that elusive house—and took physical actions to convince my mom that she meant it.

In this chapter, I offer two kinds of advice. The first set might help you when your person is about to embark on a moment of extreme agitation, and the second set might help you prevent getting there in the first place. Both sets of advice are founded on the deeply seated emotional attachment to some notion of home.

What I wish I could have told my daughter, and what I wish I had known myself, is that when our person demands to go home, the request is not literal. Instead, the request signals a need for comfort, security, or joy associated with home. When a person with dementia experiences a negative emotional state—because of uncomfortable clothing, a change in schedule, a change in scenery, physical discomfort brought about by illness or medication, or some other factor—they crave comfort and safety. This may cause their desire for *home* to kick in. They may shout for home, demand it, and try to go find it for themselves, but what they're really looking for is safety, security, control, and love.

When your person expresses a desire to go home, consider the request as metaphorical instead of literal. Consider reframing their request in the privacy of your mind: they're not asking for a location—they're asking for an emotional state. This is good news, because even though you can't bring them back in time, you can likely channel some of the emotional security they're looking for.

Emotional security is an odd thing. When we give it to small children, we might say something like, "We'll get gas in the car and then go home." We use logic. We use if/then statements. The child can see the sense of the time progression, and they look for the landmarks. *Here come our bags, then we get the car, and then we go home.* But our person with dementia might not respond to logic particularly well. Their brains find concepts of time and sequences tricky and unreliable. When we tell a child that a building no longer exists, they believe us. When we tell our person that there is no building, they might not believe us.

If I could go back in time and talk to myself while I was in the airport with my mother, I would say, "Tell her what she wants to hear." I would tell myself to be less reluctant to lie to her. I could have said, "Yes, mom. We're going to your mom's house." Furthermore, while waiting for those bags, I would have embarked on a conversation about her own mom. What would they do when mom got home? Who else would be there? I would have leaned on my mom's emotional attachment to her mom to distract her from her current discomfort.

Additionally, I would tell myself to bring other people on board earlier. When mom heard my brother's voice reassuring her, she calmed down. My daughter fumbled into a similar solution when taking care of my mom. When grandma wanted to go home, and was unconsolably crying, my daughter called her uncle and asked where the house was. She told her grandma that they'd take a road trip, and because my daughter had talked to her uncle in front of her grandma, grandma believed her. Thankfully, my mother forgot about the road trip before my daughter needed to load her and her two small kids into the car and traipse around New England.

In the process of writing this book, my daughter and I discussed this series of events. I told her that I shouldn't have taken my mom on that trip. I should have kept her home, away from the triggers that led to behaviors that scared everyone. My daughter reminded me that we didn't know until that trip how far my mom's dementia had progressed, and she also reminded me that my mom had enjoyed large swaths of that trip. Maybe we should be happy that my mom had one last trip where she got to do one of her favorite things—visit her kids, grandkids, and great grandkids. My daughter reminded me that I should be kind to myself—which seems like familiar advice.

Parkinson's and Lewy body disease often come with a phenomenon called time-shifting. Your person with dementia might feel absolutely convinced that it's time to pick the kids up from school—despite the fact that the kids now have kids themselves. Your person might be convinced that it's time to go to the airport or the train station. In their minds, they are living in another time and place. They may not recognize current technology or even themselves in the mirror. Time-shifting may come and go. As I discovered the hard way, researchers report that the most effective interventions include sensory engagement and positive distractions.[2]

After I had become more familiar with ways to keep my mom happy as her dementia progressed, she was visiting my home. We went out to feed the birds, but when we came back, she didn't recognize the house. "We can't go in there," she said. "We don't know who lives there." In the past, I might have tried to correct her, to tell her that I, in fact, lived there. But instead, I told her that she was right. We turned around, fed more birds, and came back. She had forgotten her concern about the house and, this time, walked right in without stress.

In summary, this is the advice I have for you. First, avoid arguing with or correcting your person. If they are convinced that they need to go to their mother's house, telling them that their mother is gone will not help. Telling them that their kids graduated twenty years ago won't help. Logic and time aren't friends of your person anymore.

Second, don't be afraid to lie to them. It's okay to tell them that you all are heading to mom's house now. Take that walk to the school bus or that ride to the airport. Make plans for a road trip that you won't actually make. They will likely experience another time shift or forget what you were doing. Third, don't be afraid to bring other people on board. You built a team in chapter 1. Lean on those people now. Call your brother or your neighbor or your friend and ask them to help. Sometimes hearing another familiar voice will calm them. Sometimes having another person corroborate your story is helpful. At the very least, they can make you a cup of tea when the moment has passed.

My last piece of advice is this: become a sleuth. What was your person doing just before things went south? For example, whenever my mom was triggered to find home, things went sideways quickly. She'd climb fences and run through truck stops. I started keeping notes on what we were doing just before that. I realized that taking her to unfamiliar places—like the airport, visiting my house, traveling to a new destination, traveling in a stranger's car, or even coming into her own home after a tiring outing—made an outburst more likely. When she also endured physical or emotional stress, an outburst became very likely. This realization allowed me to know when she needed extra care. I could help things by staying close to her, taking her hand, and ensuring her with comforting words that everything was okay—and we were going home. I never again left her standing in the baggage claim while I went off searching for luggage.

In this section I've tried to give you tools that might help while you and your person are in crisis, and these tools lean heavily on the emotional security associated with the concept of *home*. In the next section, I'll try to give you tools that help you make your person's current home more of a safe haven, more of a place that they crave for comfort and security, so that when your person wants to go home, their current dwelling is the place that they crave.

THE PHYSICAL HOME: MAKE THE STRUCTURE SAFE AND COMFORTABLE FOR YOUR PERSON

Before we can discuss ways to make a home feel homey, we need to discuss safety. Of adults over sixty-five, 90 percent report that they prefer to stay in their own homes as they age.[3] People with dementia are no different, and there are benefits to aging in place. These include preserving independence, health benefits, maintaining identity, preserving community and social connections, and savings money.[4] Seniors, even those with dementia, have significantly improved quality of life when they can age in place.[5] However, living at home with dementia requires some special modifications, and the following section describes some interventions that may help you keep your person with dementia living at home as long as possible.

Plan early: Modifications to stairways, bathrooms, bedrooms, and kitchens are best made before the need arises. Once a health crisis such as a broken hip or a stroke presents itself, home alterations become trickier and more expensive, and often drive people to nursing facilities earlier than would have been necessary. When modifying a home, or shopping for a new one, try to keep three things in mind: (1) fall avoidance, (2) fall mitigation, and (3) access to bathrooms, bedrooms, and kitchens. Specifically, consider these modifications to avoid early admittance to a care facility.

- **Access:** People require *stairless* access to their kitchen, bath, and bedroom. We also need to be able to enter and exit our homes without the use of stairs. This might mean adding ramps at a front or back door, even if they are just to accommodate a single step. Also consider providing clear traffic paths through your home. This might mean moving furniture and clutter to open critical areas. Could you move from your driveway to all the key rooms in your house in a wheelchair or with a walker?
- **Doors:** After you've considered the stair issue, now you might want to consider your doorways. Could a wheelchair fit through your front

door and through the key rooms in your house? How would a person with a walker fare? You may need to widen your doorways.

- **Kitchen:** As discussed in earlier chapters, contributing to your community is good for your mental health. If you cannot warm your own coffee or make your own soup, you might begin to feel depressed. To prevent this, consider what it would be like to use your kitchen with a walker or a wheelchair. Appliances should be located at an accessible height. Consider lowering the counter or primary work surface for food preparation. Could you reach the microwave from a wheelchair?
- **Bathroom:** Consider replacing the bathtub with a walk-in shower for safe entry and exit. You could install safety bars at the tub, sink, and toilet. Also consider adding a bathtub bench for sitting during showering and a handheld shower nozzle to make washing easier.
- **Flooring:** When using carpet, consider a short-nap pile; tripping is easier with longer naps, and shorter naps facilitate the use of walkers and wheelchairs. Try to avoid throw rugs, especially on hard-surface floors, since they cause tripping. Loose rugs promote tripping, and patterns may contribute to hallucinations. See if you can avoid stone, marble, or brick floors. They become dangerously slippery when wet and are unkind to heads, knees, and hips when you fall on them.
- **Smart technology:** Assistive technology can significantly make aging in place safer and often requires no permanent changes to the house. They can range from monitoring medical alerts to security systems. See chapter 8, "Technology for Dementia."

By reducing the number of potential dangers, hazards, and environmental stressors in your home, you are creating a dwelling in which your person with dementia will be safe. Toward that end, you've adapted your home so that the floors are less likely to be the cause of a fall. You've reduced clutter and thereby reduced items that might trip someone. You've made sure that you can fit wheelchairs through the doors, and you've made your home stair-free. I discuss furnishings in chapter 5, but we still have more things to discuss here. In the following section, I will provide some ideas regarding how we can make the insides of our houses more supportive for those with dementia.

Taking advantage of the disease: Cognitive mapping concerns our orientation, spatial understanding, and our ability to navigate the environment. As dementia progresses, this ability diminishes. Difficulties in navigation and recognizing one's own home or spaces within their home are common symptoms of dementia. This means that people with dementia increasingly depend on visual elements.[6] A recent review[7] found that because people with dementia can't see subtle differences in color, they eat better with tableware that contrasts with the table and they find doors more easily when frames contrast with walls. This same phenomenon could be used to mask exit doors or doorknobs, effectively preventing exit attempts. Consider finding brightly colored flatware and dishes and setting them on light-colored tablecloths. You might paint doors that you want your person to find in colors that contrasts the walls, and camouflage the doors you're prefer they would ignore.

Because people with dementia lose their ability to interpret the environment, you can help your person by adding more cues, which enhances memory by providing support for encoding and retrieval, creating less demand to process information. Wang and Lu[8] report, for instance, that clearer toilet signage resulted in better continence. Consider finding obvious art that designates a room as appropriate for bodily functions. Signs and images in kitchens, bathing areas, and bedrooms might also be helpful.

People with dementia struggle with large, open spaces and with large groups. As you modify your home, consider reducing your reliance on the larger rooms, keeping your smaller rooms reduced of clutter, and keeping your group size small.

Walls: Walls can provide enormous canvases in one's home. Dementia-friendly environments use this canvas to enhance sensory stimulation, mitigate disruptive behavior, and provide remanence therapy. For example, a wall with a shelf of exciting objects will encourage the person to pick up the object out of curiosity and delight. You know your person. Consider adding elements from their youth. Were they farmers? Consider old farming implements. My husband always enjoyed architectural tools, so I had a shelf filled with slide rulers, pens, and paper. A shelf filled with hats and scarves might be fun for other people. Simple blackboards and message boards are a terrific low-tech option to engage in communication. Large magnetic walls with cards, words, and pictures can be engaging and fun. Clocks and calendars are interactive communication and can be strategically placed for prime viewing. Be prepared to remove items if your person finds them upsetting. My mom became vexed with calendars and clocks. For additional discussions about interventions based on art, artifacts, and nostalgic items, see chapter 5, "Furnishings Matter."

Ceilings: Ceilings are often forgotten as intervention opportunities as they are generally not part of the field of vision. However, ceilings play a crucial role in how one feels and interacts with home, and people perceive the size of the space by what they see below the ceiling. High ceilings feel more spacious; lower ceilings feel cozier. You might not be able to change your ceiling height, but you can affect the way your person interacts with it. If your person becomes bedridden, even temporarily, consider putting up pictures and funny images or projecting a slide show. There are a number of affordable constellation projectors, sky projectors, and projectors where you insert your own family photos.

Flooring: Flooring is one of the most challenging materials in homes. For cleanability, many consider hard-surface floors most appropriate. However, visual misperception from glare or from wet floors can cause serious falls; even dry hard-surface floors can be slippery, and falls on hard surfaces produce more severe injuries. People still fall on carpeted floors, but carpet tends to cause less severe injuries. Carpets have no glare, and that may reduce the number of falls. Additionally, vacuuming carpeted floors is less disruptive than washing hard-surface floors because you don't need to close the room. Carpeting mitigates airborne bacteria, while hard surfaces have higher airborne bacteria. Most homes use combinations of both, maximizing the benefits while minimizing concerns in specific areas.

Temperature: Proper room temperatures can help keep seniors comfortable and healthy. As we age, our ability to thermoregulate decreases, which means that we cannot rely so heavily on our metabolism to keep us comfortable. The ideal room temperature for the elderly is 78 degrees, ranging from 65 to 78 degrees depending on your person. The temperature should never exceed 80 degrees because as we age, we have difficulty maintaining proper hydration; overly warm rooms promote dehydration, which promotes illness. Room temperature should never drop below 65 because hypothermia may occur, promoting illness.

Proper temperatures promote health by impacting memory, the heart and lungs, the immune system, and comfort. Dealing with heat and cold is uncomfortable, and this discomfort can quickly turn to pain; and, as we've discussed, pain and discomfort may lead to outbursts. I suggest that you consider monitoring the temperature so that you know when the temperature goes up or down to dangerous levels. Smart technology can help, and some electric companies offer discounts to people who use it. (See chapter 8, "Technology for Dementia.") Consider inspecting your windows and doors for spaces or cracks and repair them. You will keep you and your person more comfortable and lower your energy bill. Also consider preparing for power outages with backup plans. Do you have a generator or someplace to go if you lose power during an extreme weather event?

Humidity: Because our ability to thermoregulate declines with age, environmental humidity, like temperature, requires more attention as we age. Humidity levels should range between 35 percent and 60 percent. Low humidity levels can cause skin irritations and the transmission of viruses. High humidity promotes the growth of bacteria and dust mites, which can lead to unpleasant odors and respiratory irritation.

To keep an eye on humidity levels, you can use a hygrometer, a device that measures indoor humidity. Smart technology can also help. (See chapter 8, "Technology for Dementia.") If your heating/AC system doesn't automatically control humidity, using dehumidifiers during humid seasons and humidifiers during dry seasons can help you maintain appropriate indoor humidity levels.

Air quality: As we age, we become more susceptible to the effects of airborne pollutants. Contaminants like dust, mold spores, and smoke particulates from volatile organic compounds (VOCs) or building materials are more likely to irritate our lungs and health as we age. High carbon dioxide levels are also unhealthy. Indoor pollutants can damage the cardiovascular, endocrine, immune, nervous, and respiratory systems.[9] Pain and irritation increase the likelihood of outbursts in our person.

High-efficiency particulate air (HEPA) filters capture airborne pollutants, removing 99 percent of dust, pollen, mold, bacteria, and other airborne particles. Many home heating and air conditioning systems can be adapted with a HEPA filter, and portable HEPA filters are available at lower costs. HEPA vacuum cleaners are also available. Carbon dioxide monitors, like smoke detectors, are inexpensive and easily installed. I recommend that you check your stove, air conditioner, and furnace filters seasonally. Weather permitting, natural ventilation— open doors and windows—can also improve indoor air.

Clean hands: Handwashing can help mitigate the transmission of infectious diseases. Dirty hands from toileting, personal care, eating, and other activities of daily living often lead to bacteria transmission. Regular manicures that help keep nails short and clean are a human-centric approach to good hygiene and prevent bacteria buildup under nails. Handwashing before and after meals, and toileting, upon entering home are also necessary. Regular handwashing is also essential to maintain good health. People with dementia find it challenging to complete handwashing tasks, and it is difficult to remember the activity or understand the process, and that they must comply. A caregiver must gently coach them through the job.

The clean house: I recommend that you wash knobs, handles, and frequently touched surfaces. Maybe your person can help. Microbiologically contaminated surfaces can serve as a reservoir for pathogens and facilitate disease transmission.

Transitioning into a Care Home

There may come a time when aging in place is no longer appropriate. Often this point comes on the heels of another dramatic change. Your person might have fallen and broken a hip. Your person's caregiver might have died or become unable to provide care. You, the caregiver, might just become overwhelmed. No magic formula, schedule, or phase can tell you when or if the time is right. Many caregivers are devoted to keeping their loved ones at home as long as possible. Perhaps they have promised their person that they would never move them to a nursing home. However, there are many reasons why moving to a care facility is not only necessary but the correct thing to do. It is often one of the most challenging decisions we face.

Caregivers often struggle with this decision, feel guilt, wait too long, and compromise their own health. I endured a stress-related heart attack while caring for my late husband. Sometimes the decision involves less drama. Needing to travel for work, my husband and I placed my father-in-law, with mid-stage Alzheimer's, in a care facility for a week. When we went to pick him up, he suggested that he stay permanently. He liked his new friends.

Researchers[10] have pinpointed these common reasons for admittance to care facilities:

- Your person requires high-tech nursing care. This might include medical devices, equipment, or unique treatments such as intravenous medication.

- You cannot accommodate your person's mobility. Your person uses a wheelchair and you cannot lift, bathe, or provide other activities of daily living.
- Your person uses disruptive behavior. My mom's nighttime elopement became unmanageable, disrupting the neighborhood and her safety.
- You, the caregiver, might be in declining health or growing too old. My grandfather, at ninety-eight, was taking care of my grandmother, ninety-six, with dementia.
- Your person might enter the late stages of dementia where issues such as incontinence, an inability to recognize you, or an inability to communicate mean that level of care needed exceeds what you can provide.

The conversation: Discuss care options with your loved one before the disease advances. It is always comforting to know their wishes, and it may relieve your guilt, if that's an emotion you contend with. Try to remember that your mental and physical health play a significant role in this decision. If you can't take care of your person any longer, you should allow yourself to consider alternatives. Most caregivers experience less burden and less tension following the transition, which is good for their health, as discussed in the first chapter. Your caregiving responsibilities do not end when your loved one moves to a care facility. They just change, including a larger care team with a new home model. Your loved one will need your caregiving support, especially after moving.

Consider finding a suitable care home before a crisis occurs, maybe even before the disease progresses too far. This may allow you to locate the right place for you and your person. A thoughtful choice made by two people helps make the transition less difficult, and if by the time the disease progresses your person does not remember your joint decision, try to remember that it is the nature of the disease, not your person.

Many dementia "home" options exist. Memory care options are found within retirement communities, assisted living, village concepts, and skilled nursing homes. They offer various services, including super-vised care and housing. The Continuing Care Retirement Community (CCRC) also provides a continuum of care—independent living, as-sisted living, skilled nursing, and memory care—within one campus or establishment.

These diverse options also have many variations. There are also in-novative models for senior housing, including the greenhouse model, co-housing, and pocket neighborhoods. Each of these models may also have variations that focus on innovations such as universal design, com-munity, and wellness, such as the WELL Building Standard, a building certification that focuses on people's health and well-being, and the Green House models. The Edan Alternative and Planetree models focus on patient-centered experience. Given the long-term nature of demen-tia, lasting up to twenty-plus years, a person may transition through many of these models, selecting homes and services that best meet their current needs. Maybe find time to explore which of these options ex-ist near you and which best serves the needs of both your person and yourself before the disease advances too far.

Making a care facility feel like home: Now that you have found the right place for your loved one and are planning the move, consider what can be done to achieve the feeling of home. The best tool is your knowl-edge. You know your person—their likes, dislikes, fears, and delights. You and your team can transform the facility's resident room into their new home.

When you are preparing your person's new space, consider taking some time to evaluate the house they are leaving. What did they love best about it? How can you incorporate the treasured elements into the new home? You can have these conversations with your person before the disease progresses. Chat about treasured items and the stories behind them. These old favorites represent personal stories and evoke memories. This is not the time to go out and buy new things; even broken or old items are relevant, as they invoke deep memories that are hard to otherwise access. This awareness will help determine what things can best support them in their next home.

Very personal items—her hairbrush, prayer book, favorite teacup, or coffee mug, things that you remember lying around forever—each of these should be part of the move. They make a big difference in retaining identity. Maxcine had a teapot collection, but her favorite was a little blue one with a broken cover, and she used it daily. Even with the fractured top, the little teapot found a perfect spot on her table in her new home.

Photos, photo collages, and photo albums of family, life's trips, and life's significant events are powerful tools that help keep memories alive. Years ago, Maxcine had created a large photo collage of her family, mounted on an antique headboard. We brought it to her new apartment and placed it in a prominent location. It became a great conversation starter for visitors and staff. Everyone loved it, and it helped the team identify with Maxcine and get to know her personally.

Bedding, blankets, pillows, and snuggly dolls are nurturing and provide great comfort when sleeping in a new place. Again, this is not the time for fresh new linens. Old, recognizable, soft blankets, especially pillows with familiar smells, can help calm. My grandmother was unable to sleep and anguished over her tiny single bed without room for her husband, exclaiming she could never sleep here! We brought her old pillow from home, and she cried joyfully and could sleep comfortably.

Putting a loved one into a care facility may be one of the most difficult decisions a family will have to make. Initially, life can be different and overwhelming, but it is not the end. A person can continue to feel loved and cared for and join other residents in social activities. They can continue friendship and family connections.

CONCLUSION

Homes are both structural buildings and emotional states. Our people with dementia easily confuse them, and knowing that can help you in both times of emergency and times of peace, when emergencies can be prevented. You can modify your current home to best support your person with dementia, considering safety, cues to room functions, and the physical environment. If and when your person needs to move to a care facility, you can bring emotional home elements to their new space to ease the transition.

5

Furnishings Matter

My in-laws from Florida moved in with us. It happened on a visit where we found his mother dying of cancer and his father in mid-stage Alzheimer's. While my husband and I had discussed an eventuality of them living with us, we never imagined it would happen during a weekend visit.

Since we were traveling by plane, we returned to Virginia with only their clothing and a few personal effects. Once home, we modified our family room and guest room into an apartment, hoping they'd feel comfortable. They had their own space: a bedroom, a kitchenette, a family room with a TV, and their own access to the patio and backyard.

After a whirlwind of doctor visits and trips to the store, we settled into a routine. Following dinner, we would relax together with a movie or conversation. However, his dad wouldn't join us on the sofa. He claimed he would break it and would only sit on the dining room chair, which was too hard and uncomfortable. After sitting a short time, he would become restless. He would wander and become agitated, as if looking for something.

Initially, we thought he no longer enjoyed TV or found the program we selected uninteresting. We then remembered that he had his favorite easy chair where he'd sit to watch television and talk with guests. Because we had left furnishings behind, we no longer had his favorite chair.

To solve this, we purchased another that was very similar in color and design. When we told him we had found his old chair, he happily sat and watched TV with us.

As dementia took hold of my husband, he had a different reaction to a personal chair. Joe had never retreated to a chair to watch TV; he preferred to snuggle with me on the sofa. Even when we had guests, he preferred the sofa. Furthermore, his architectural aesthetic did not include a recliner.

On Joe's dementia journey, he would retreat to the daybed for a nap when he was tired or upset. I took this as a sign that he needed a recliner. I found what I thought was the perfect chair. It didn't look like a recliner and would have met his pre-dementia ideals for aesthetics. However, he refused to use it. When the chair was suggested for a nap, he'd say, "This is Barbara's chair," and head off to the daybed for his nap.

If I could go back in time and speak to my earlier self, I'd tell her: if your person has a favorite furniture item, respect it, and keep it with them throughout their journey. If they don't have this attachment, don't force it on them.

MEET YOUR FURNITURE

Designers define *furnishings* as household items that appoint the home. They include equipment, appliances, window coverings, hard furnishings like tables and chairs, and soft furnishings like blankets and toys. Furnishings might seem utilitarian and mundane, lacking relevance to dementia care, but poorly planned furnishings can pose health risks, cause accidents, and contribute to loneliness. Furthermore, because people form attachments to furnishings, as my father-in-law demonstrated, they can provide a path toward positive intervention for our people with dementia. This chapter considers furnishings as potential tools for interventions, improving tools we already have and providing new ones that might make our lives easier.

FUNCTIONAL FURNISHINGS

Furnishings have three components that are worth our consideration as we try to support our people with dementia. These components include comfort, safety, and placement. In the following sections, I'll describe how to maximize the intervention potential of furnishings by considering each of the components.

Comfort: As we age and mobility declines, we spend much more time sitting. Sitting upright requires that muscles work against gravity to hold a correct posture. As we age, the muscles become weaker, and we may slouch. Poor posture leads to health risks, including chest, lung, and urinary tract infections. Physical comfort, always vital, becomes something that needs to be planned. Furnishings can help.

Researchers define *ergonomic* as a characteristic of any work-related item that was specifically designed for maximum comfort and efficiency. Ergonomic chairs facilitate upright posture while providing lumbar support. They allow the necks of people using them to remain in a relaxed and neutral position, feet to remain flat on the floor, and arms to rest parallel to the floor.

We've learned from the workplace that good ergonomics can make seating more comfortable, and we have evidence that good ergonomics reduce the risk of chronic spine, joint, and muscle problems, and that ergonomic seating can reduce the frequency and intensity of pain for people already having these issues. By allowing people to think about things other than their bodies, we have improved their efficiency in the workplace. Furthermore, we can bring that knowledge into our homes to support our people with dementia.

Supporting your person with ergonomic seating starts with observation. Does your person struggle to reach items, or do they have difficulty sitting or standing? If so, maybe their seating isn't working for them and ergonomic adjustments may help. Ergonomic seating uses four metrics: (1) arms and arm height, (2) back height, (3) seat depth and seat height, and (4) cushion construction. In this section, I will discuss each.

- **Arms and arm height:** As we age, we rely on the arms of our seats to provide aid as we sit and stand. Arms ideally should be 11 inches or more taller than the seat. When considering arms on sofa seating, low arms and armless sofas may offer little support to your person. If your person manages to sit on such a sofa, they may feel stuck when it's time to stand. Try to avoid low-armed and no-armed sofas. On the other hand, sofas with overly high arms might prevent our people from reaching adjacent end tables, so try to avoid the overly tall-armed sofas too. Seating in the kitchens and dining is worth a note. If your chair arms fit under your tabletops, your person can get closer to the table, reducing spills and messes.
- **Back height:** Ergonomic seating recommends that the back height of a seat support the sitter's head and should be at least 18 inches tall. If your person uses a low-backed chair either as a sofa or for dining, and you see that they have developed a habit of leaning, you might consider changing the chair to something with a higher back.
- **Seat depth:** Seat depth should be narrow, so feet can reach the floor. Researchers find the 19-inch seat depth works best for most people. In general, elderly people don't do well with large, deep, sectional sofas. While families, children, and dogs like to snuggle up on them, people who are a bit frail might be uncomfortable and helpless in the same setting. Try to ensure that your person with dementia can sit on a sofa with their feet on the floor and have a sofa arm to assist, to maximize safety and comfort.
- **Seat height:** Like arm height, seat height supports people as they sit and stand. People with dementia can struggle with stability, and appropriate seat height can help. A seat height of 17 to 18 inches is best for most people because it provides a landing spot that is not too low to the ground and a seat that is not too hard to leave, especially with appropriate arm rests. When sitting, a person's feet should sit flat on the floor.
- **Cushion construction:** Cushion construction refers to the softness or firmness of the seat. Soft cushions increase comfort but do not support transitioning from sitting to standing. Firm cushions work well for short-term sitting, like at meals, but your person can get uncomfortable if they remain sitting on them for long periods. Consider softer cushions for chairs where you'd like your person to linger.

- **More on cushions:** Pillows are a great assistant to compensate for seating shortcomings. Consider adding a pillow at you person's back to decrease the seat depth. You can put a pillow in the corners of a seat, even on a sofa, to help your person stand. Adding a pillow under your person might increase their comfort—and their ability to see.

Safety: The second component one might consider when using furnishings as an intervention in dementia is safety. Safe furnishings minimize the probability of trips and falls, and they also minimize disease spread. This section discusses both aspects of safety.

In the section above on ergonomics, I suggested that ergonomic chairs and seating were not only comfortable but safe. I would like to reiterate that point here. In properly adjusted chairs, not only are muscles, lungs, and hearts supported, but seat heights, arm rest heights, and chair back heights reduce the probability of tripping and falling when transitioning from sitting to standing and vice versa.

Additional safety measures exist for furniture. Wobbling furniture isn't helpful, no matter how beloved. Also, sharp-cornered tables can cause bruises, and bruises can lead to blood clots. Consider fixing problematic furniture items, moving them into storage, or giving them away. Now is not the time in your life to compromise safety.

Our people with dementia may spend much of their time sitting. They may spill drinks, drop food, or struggle with incontinence. This can become a safety issue because the bacteria associated with food, drink, and bodily fluids will breed. The seating can become soiled, dirty, or smelly. This may trigger disruptive behavior, and it may discourage guests from lingering.

Furnishings that are easy to clean support caregiving. Using a moisture-blocking fabric can protect fabrics from food, drinks, and incontinence. Vinyl, waterproof fabric, moisture barrier pads, or fabric with a built-in moisture barrier prevent bacterial buildup in filling materials that can't be cleaned or disinfected. You can purchase such a fabric to place over an existing seat at a very low cost. Consider purchasing extras so you have a fresh one when the dirty one is in the laundry.

Placement: The third component one might consider when using furnishings as an intervention in dementia is furniture placement. The social environment, such as the living room, family room, and dining room, provides a physical and personal place to participate in family and social events. The layout of furnishings contributes to safety and can facilitate social interactions.

Let's consider safety first. You might ask yourself if the room is organized in such a way so that people can move around without knocking their shins and knees. For example, a coffee table with legs that curve outward can become a tripping hazard. Is there enough room between the sofa and table for your person to walk? Researchers find that 30 to 34 inches of clear space on the front and side of chairs provides enough space to safely sit and stand.[1]

Similarly, placing furniture too far away from a natural landing spot can generate trouble. An end table located too far from the sofa might cause a fall or trigger disruptive behavior. Can you reach that beverage on the end table easily when sitting on your sofa? If your person needs to get into and out of a wheelchair, can you rearrange your furniture so that you both have enough space for this activity?

Lastly, consider positioning furniture so that your person can lean on it for balance. A sturdy bureau or table can—and will—act as a handrail. But when your person hangs on that bookshelf to steady themselves, will it stay in place? Many types of chairs and other furnishings have castors. You might check that they're locked because a chair that rolls away as your person tries to sit can act as a hazard. Consider ensuring that you only have sturdy, not wobbly, well-anchored items in your living space before your person gets too far on their dementia journey.

People with dementia can struggle to distinguish items that share features. Your person may find it challenging to distinguish a wooden chair from a wooden table, particularly if they're placed next to each other and have a similar height. They may sit on the table; if the table isn't sturdy or well anchored, it may facilitate a fall. Can you make your table and chair look more different, perhaps by changing a color or location?

The last point I'd like to make on this topic concerns clutter rather than furnishings. Because people with dementia cannot easily distinguish one object from another, reducing your clutter might make their world easier to navigate. If only one item on a table looks like a lamp, your person is more likely to use the lamp correctly. Clutter can become a safety issue too. Magazine stacks, small piles of backpacks, books, and shoes, dishes, and laptops tend to pile up, and they can become a tripping hazard, especially if you tend to stack these things on stairs or the floor. You may want to reorganize your home so that all such items have a place where you can store them out of sight. Many big falls are caused by small items.

Now that you've made your living space safe, maybe you can adjust it so that it better supports social interactions. Seating can help. If your person can see and hear visitors, they may be more inclined to sit and chat. Also consider your visitors here. Friendly seating allows enough space but isn't so far spaced that people struggle to hear. Additionally, everyone likes clean space and space that is easy to enter and exit.

On a visit with my grandmother, we passed her friend sitting on a bench and invited her to lunch. "I'd love to, dears, but I can't— I'm stuck here."

"What do you mean?" I asked.

Unable to get off her seat, she reached up to me. I had to help her stand because the bench had no arms or back. If we hadn't come along, she would have missed the opportunity for social engagement.

ASSISTIVE FURNISHINGS

Now that we've discussed the comfort, safety, and placement of furniture, I'd like to introduce the idea of furnishings that support furniture: assistive furnishings. Assistive furnishings are designed to be used while coupled with standard furniture to support specific tasks. They can be great problem solvers.

The first type of assistive furnishing I'd like to introduce is the *tray*. Trays come in two main types: the kind you clamp onto another piece of furniture, or the type you slide over another piece of furniture. For example, you can clamp a tray onto a recliner, a coffee table, or even a dining table to adjust the height. You can also attach them to sofas, chairs, beds, and baths, giving yourself an adjacent surface for food, meds, or accessories. Some trays look like end tables but have legs only on one side, so that you can slide them over a chair, sofa, or bed. Some tray tables have adjustable swivel mechanisms to move them out of the way when unneeded, and others offer stand-assist handles. A cup holder and newspaper/magazine saddles attached to the side of the seating can provide comfort and convenience.

The second type of assistive furnishing I'd like to introduce are sit-stand support products. These work much like canes but are linked with furniture, providing steady support to people getting in and out of seating. The frame fits neatly under the sofa, chair, and bed, and it has comfortable grips for a secure hold. Some have attached trays. These are easily available from Amazon and other retailers.

Chairs

We discussed ergonomics in seating above, but in this section, I'd like to discuss specific chair types. While all furnishings matter, many people have a personal connection to a specific chair, and as dementia progresses, your person might spend an increasing amount of time in that chair. The chair may serve as your person's ultimate nest. If this sounds like your person, the following section might help you make your person's chair a little safer or more comfortable.

The wheelchair: If your person spends much time in a wheelchair, you might be able to improve its comfort level. Sometimes the armrests can be upgraded so that they can fold down, allowing the chair to get close to tables. Foldable armrests also facilitate easy transfer. You might also be able to splurge on the seat cushion. Some chairs have adjustable arm and seat heights. See the ergonomics section on how to adjust those heights. Lumbar support cushions increase comfort and facilitate good posture. Accessories like heating pads, cup holders, and saddle bags can make life more comfortable and convenient.

The recliner: If your person loves a recliner, they can safely operate it in the early and sometimes the middle stages of dementia. These chairs often support those with mobility issues since they have a rise-assist that helps people exit the chair. Also, the chair can be equipped with safety sensors if you have pets or small children in your life. On the downside, in the later stages of dementia, these chairs may become a risk as the controls become confusing and potentially triggering.

High-back chairs: High-back chairs can comfortably provide head support. Some have adjustable backs, and you can see how to adjust them ergonomically if you read the section above. Wing chairs impede side vision and hearing and don't facilitate social interactions. I recommend that you avoid these. If you're using high-back chairs as dining chairs, you might consider determining whether they are both stable and moveable for your person.

The rocking chair: As with the recliner, the rocking chair has costs and benefits. The rocker is often a favorite because it creates a calming effect for those with dementia. The rocking motion stimulates the vestibular canal in the ear, supporting the sense of balance and calm. Consider a stable platform-type rocker to maximize the safety of those entering and exiting the chair. Rockers present a fall risk and require personal assistance when getting into and out of them.

Fabrics

Fabrics can be used to highlight or obscure furnishings for your person. For instance, if you want to invite your person with dementia to sit in a particular place, you can increase the probability of that happening not only with placement but by making it visible. Very simple patterns or no patterns make it easiest for most people with dementia to see and understand. Large-scale prints can confuse your person to the point where they don't see the chair as a chair. Multiple patterns and high contrast on a single chair can also confuse. People with dementia tend to see patterns with small dots and specks as something to pick at, distracting them from sitting. Unicolor fabrics that contrast with the surrounding colors are the most likely to draw your person to the chair and invite them to use it appropriately. If your current chair has a disruptive pattern, consider covering it with a throw or slipcover.

The Bedroom

The bedroom is important because we all spend a lot of time in ours and because, as the disease progresses, your person may spend increasing amounts of time in there. In this section, I'd like to discuss the furnishings and layout associated with this space. Bedroom furnishings and layout can support a good night's sleep for your person—and yourself—and reduce agitation and incontinence in your person. You might not be able to change the layout of your current bedroom, but if you move your person to a care facility, layout may be in your control. Whether you are adjusting a current bedroom or setting up a new one, this section might be helpful.

The bed: If you can, try to locate the bed so that it provides a view of the toilet. Seeing the toilet while lying in bed will help your person with incontinence. If the bedroom does not include a bathroom, you might add floor lights and handrails directly from the bedroom to the bathroom. Placing a bathroom sign with an arrow to the bathroom down the hall might help your person. Seeing the bathroom or the sign will help them recall why they woke up and what they need to do.

While hospital beds are not the norm in homes, if your person has one and objects to it, consider adding a residential-style headboard. Can you attach your old one to the new bed? Now isn't the time to buy new bedding. Try to bring as much of their original bedding, mattress, and pillows as possible. The attention to this detail will help the transition from home to a care facility and may reduce sleep problems.

The wardrobe: The wardrobe or closet should be small and simple. Large closets are too overwhelming and become confusing when people are selecting clothing. If you are adjusting your existing closet for your person, consider removing all but the most basic clothing and footwear choices since people with dementia find it challenging to distinguish between things. You may wish to lock the door if your loved one mistakes the closet door for the bathroom door.

The dresser: While you should be able to see the bathroom from the bed, try to position the dresser directly opposite from the bed if your person has a television. You can mount the television above the dresser to provide good viewing from the bed. If you aren't using a television in the bedroom, you have more flexibility with the location of the dresser.

The personal chair: If you can, try to position the chair with good sightlines to the door, outdoor window, television, and bathroom. If your person can feel comfortable in their chair, they may use it more, and you can maximize comfort by maximizing views. A table with a task lamp could be placed adjacent to it, and an optional desk is helpful for computer use and family communications.

Storage: Storage includes dressers, chests of drawers, night tables, and bookshelves. People with dementia may struggle to remember the location of their things. Storage furniture should be easy to open and contain only a few options. Adding labels such as "Socks" with a picture of socks on the drawer front can be helpful and extend the period of independence. If you are selecting furniture, look for rounded, soft edges. If handles contrast in color from the door or drawer, your person with dementia can more easily see them. You may be able to easily change out your current handles for those that contrast more in color.

The Bathroom

In chapter 2, "A Sense of Place," I provided some suggestions for reducing disruptive behavior while helping your person with the bathroom. Here, I expand on that conversation, including design elements that might both reduce disruptive behavior and improve safety. Bathrooms frequently contribute to falls, loss of dignity, and disruptive behaviors for people with dementia, so you might find this additional discussion helpful.

To use the bathroom, your person needs to find it. While dementia might make this challenging, you can help. For instance, you could add a charming bathroom sign on the door to easily identify the room. A light sensor at the bathroom entrance can also help your person identify the room. If you can manage it, your person might benefit from handrails leading from the bedroom to the bathroom. A low-tech alternative is a reflective tape to guide the path.

Once in the bathroom, there are some adjustments you can make to support your person's independence. People with dementia struggle to identify items, but we can help them by using contrasting colors. (For more on this, see chapter 7, "The Language of Color.") For example, if you swap out your white toilet seat for a red one, on your white bowl, your person might see it more easily. You can also contrast the color of your soap on your sink to visually prompt handwashing. If you use a contrasting color behind your toilet, it will become more visible to your person and reduce incontinence.

Regarding the toilet itself, a higher toilet might be helpful for those with balance, mobility, or wheelchair transfer issues. A seat that is 17 to 18 inches from the ground supports easy sitting and standing. You can obtain toilet-seat extenders rather than replacing the entire toilet. Is your flush mechanism easy to see? If not, can you swap it out for one of a contrasting color? Toilet paper that is easily seen and reached is more likely to be used. Holders that are simple are more likely to be used appropriately. Last, handrails will reduce the number of falls.

By visually displaying toiletry items such as brushes, toothpaste, shampoo, and shaving cream on shelves, rather than storing them in drawers, you will increase the probability that your person will use them, especially if you can add a backdrop to increase the contrast. People with dementia need to see what they need to use.

Regarding the tub or shower, safety is particularly important. If you have a choice, curb-less showers and tubs with open sides are the safest since your person won't have a curb to step over. Your person is more likely to use grabrails that contrast in color relative to the walls. Assistive furnishings, such as bath grab bars and tub transfer seats, can facilitate safe transfers. Bath seats and nonslip mats can also improve safety. These are sold in many places and are easy to install. Handheld showerheads can help you bathe your person but might be hard to understand if your person is still independent in the shower. Keep traditional faucets in place while your person can bathe themself.

For both your sink and your shower or tub, you may want to check that the water heater's thermostat setting is 120 degrees Fahrenheit, which prevents scalding. For both the sink and the shower, traditional and simple hardware are easiest to use. Hot and cold handles could be separate and labeled, but you might want to change them either very early in your person's dementia journey or very late in it. If you change them in the middle of the journey, your person may become confused.

THE ALCHEMY OF FURNISHINGS

Up until now, this chapter has covered ways to maximize the benefits of your furniture, focusing mainly on chairs and room layouts. Now we come to furnishings and the way we can harness their power to support our person. Beauty is often our last consideration when we find ourselves in the challenging role of caregiving. However, Julian Hughes[2] suggests that dementia care include beauty since aesthetics rely on intuition, communicating through touch, smell, and visual senses, thereby bypassing dementia-wrought brain damage.

Beauty is not standard, and aesthetic senses vary. For example, my grandmother loved Danish modern style and couldn't believe that her retirement home used traditional furnishings. She complained, "It's such a nice facility, but why do they have all that old stuff?" Luckily, we had the opportunity to use Danish modern design in her apartment. My neighbor moved into a beautiful new assisted living facility, but she hated it; it was too fancy. The utilitarian feel of the veterans' facility was more to her taste.

ART, ARTIFACTS, AND OBJECTS

Furnishings such as art contribute to the beauty within a room and can provide meaningful interventions in dementia therapy. Art interaction, or art observation, is a nonverbal activity that remains less affected by dementia than are other activities.[3] Art provides connection, satisfaction, familiarity, and joy, and art interaction is as easy as putting an appropriate image in the path of your person.[4]

What kind of art is right for your person? Research indicates that hospital patients prefer nature-based art content, and research consistently shows that by viewing nature-infused art, people enjoy reduced stress, lowered blood pressure, reduced need for pain medication, and increased trust and confidence.

However, people with dementia seem to prefer relatable family scenes and connections to home. My father-in-law, in a memory care facility, always stopped at a family painting of a kitchen scene. "Oh, mama was so good." He enjoyed this picture and connected with his home and relationships. Consider displaying art that is relatable to your person if you are in a position to do so. Also, since you know your person better than anyone, try not to remove or move favorite pieces within your home, unless you are moving your person to a care facility.

The Value of Objects

Emotional attachment, or *essentialism,* is the concept that objects are more than their physical properties. People form an attachment to objects. Most parents are keenly aware of object attachments, having driven back one hundred miles to retrieve their toddler's teddy bear left behind in a hotel room. Often, we hang on to this teddy into adulthood. We can't seem to part with it, and it has meaning, maybe symbolizing happy or safe times. These emotions don't fade in adulthood and are particularly sensitive in people with dementia. People often seek treasured objects as compensation for missing a close relationship,[5] and we can lean on this to support our people with dementia.

Memory Boxes

Touching treasured objects often deepens our attachment to it, and memory box therapy takes advantage of that. As their name implies, "memory" items—including treasures, photos, letters, keepsakes, and other small items—are artfully displayed to evoke memories of your person's life. Some are literal boxes that your person can open and contain items that can be moved and handled. Favorite scents, colognes, or perfumes might be added. Others have similar items that have been glued or otherwise attached as a display. You can create multiple memory boxes. For instance, if your person was a musician, you can frame a piece of music and place it where they can see it. Not only do memory boxes promote engagement and conversation opportunities, but they can also link your person with dementia to their own identity.[6]

Rummaging Therapy

Most people with dementia engage in some form of rummaging. They may search for something that they are unable to name in closets, drawers, and cabinets. My mother rummaged in my daughter's linen closet looking for something she said she'd know when she saw it. People with dementia often try to reassure themselves that their everyday items, including car keys, wallets, and purses, are close at hand.

One of the best interventions for rummaging is a purposefully made rummaging box. You as the caregiver are well equipped for this task because you know best which objects and artifacts your person will find interesting. For mom, I used a shopping bag rather than a box. I put her purse, wallet, keys, glasses, and cosmetic bag inside. The bag also held her travel teacup, a shopping notepad, licorice treats, socks, and a sweater. She was always ready for her outing. Sometimes when I could see her becoming antsy, I would hand her the bag and it would keep her busy until she calmed.

Rummage boxes can be a bit larger than memory boxes, and they usually work best with focused contents. For example, if your person was a knitter, you might include yarn, needles, and scissors. Your person might respond well to a toolbox containing nuts and bolts. A box of vintage toys might satisfy another person.

When your person starts to rummage in unwanted areas, consider pulling out one of your purposeful boxes and guide their focus. As you create the rummage boxes, remember to keep them safe; scissors might not be for everyone. This engagement helps them feel empowered.

Photo Albums

Photos albums, like memory boxes, can evoke memories, tie people to their identities, and promote conversations. Keep photo albums for your person to access when you are not there. This may be helpful to families and caregivers, allowing the visitor into the lives of your person with dementia. Because you love your person, you may want to give them many albums, but try to prevent these items from cluttering. One album is sufficient.

Reminiscence Therapy

During *reminiscence therapy*, a caregiver and a person with dementia share positive memories from the past to form a connection. Dementia affects short-term memory, but older memories are often accessible, and decorating with vintage décor from the period of early adulthood may allow your person to recall happy times from their past, either actively or passively. Seeing vintage items of their youth can trigger a feeling of nostalgia, a wistful sense of pleasure, and sentimentality for the past. Promoting and sharing old memories can decrease stress, boost mood, reduce agitation, and minimize disruptive behaviors.[7]

Household Vignettes

Practitioners have expanded Montessori concepts beyond early learning into memory care by using household furnishings to connect with meaningful activities. Household vignettes can engage the senses and memory to help those with dementia interact with the world around them. Opportunities to reconnect with pleasant past events and re-experience positive memories are the hallmark of the Montessori vignettes.[8]

These vignettes are like small stage sets to grab interest and offer positive distractions. Vignettes might include a sewing nook in a cozy corner with a comfortable chair, a basket of colorful yarn balls, a knitted blanket, and a button box. The yarn balls may not be powerful enough to call forth the memory of knitting, but the creation of a vignette invites participation. Caregivers can stage a laundry vignette with a basket of towels, napkins, or easy-to-fold linens. In the kitchen, create a unique kitchen area just for them with colorful bowls, utensils, and baking ingredients.

Seasonal Decorations

Celebrating the change of seasons and a memorable holiday can be a positive distraction. Conversely, for those with cognitive difficulties, unexpected or unusual decorations that just pop up may cause disorientation or fear. Approach the holidays with positive reassurance and engagement. Holidays and seasonal milestones are a time for celebration and create interest, joy, and pleasure. It is helpful to reminisce on past holidays. Seasonal decorations can be stimulating and meaningful. Consider using them to evoke memories of traditions.

Not all holiday decorations are appropriate. For instance, blinking lights and large displays can confuse people with dementia. Some decorations can be mistaken for edible treats, such as decorative fruits and candies, and you may want to avoid those. Your person may have a personal connection with your traditional decorations, and you may want to keep those in rotation rather than purchasing new ones.

If you can involve your person in decorating, baking, crafting, watching holiday films, or reading seasonal stories, you may be able to access old memories. Signing holiday cards, if that's part of your tradition, might be something that can generate interaction.

Doll Therapy and Attachment Behavior

When people with dementia demonstrate *attachment behavior*, they continually search for long-deceased or long-grown loved ones, or otherwise express an unmet attachment need. Sometimes they search for a child long grown, a parent long deceased, or someone else who is no longer available. While disruptive, their search indicates that they feel insecure and want comfort. Doll therapy can address this attachment need.[9]

If you think doll therapy might help, you only need a realistic-looking doll (that doesn't cry). Try leaving it where your person might find it. If your person shows interest, try not to refer to it as a doll or activities with it as *play*. If your person treats it as a real child, try to follow along. You might say something like, "Your baby looks happy today." Your person might dress, rock, pet, or care for the doll, and holding it may bring comfort to your person, thereby reducing agitation.

Depending on your person, realistic stuffed animals might provide a better way to offset disruptive behavior or agitation. Again, try not to refer to the animal as a toy or to behaviors with it as *play*. Instead, consider starting a conversation with, "Your little dog looks so happy!" Communication may expand as your person shows a greater attachment to the doll or animal.

Puppets

Puppets don't need language to express themselves and can act out empathy, love, and care. They can be silly, teach, tell stories, and problem-solve. They might be able reach your person when you can't.[10]

My father-in-law had reached a stage where he no longer responded to my voice, but I found that I could communicate with him via the help of a puppet named Fred. For example, the little monkey puppet could call my father-in-law for dinner, whereas I could not. Fred would whisper in his ear, "Daddy, please come for dinner now. We have mashed potatoes, and I know it's your favorite." Then Fred would hop down from his shoulder and follow my father-in-law into the dining room.

CONCLUSION

When you opened this chapter, you might have thought that furniture and furnishings were kind of boring and not helpful for taming the wolf at your door. I hope that I've convinced you otherwise. Not only can minor adjustments to your current furniture items help you support your person, but their placement can promote clarity in the use of space, reduce incontinence, and keep your person safe. Beyond furniture, your furnishings can help you and your person. Dolls, memory boxes, vignettes, and puppets might allow you to connect with your person after their short-term memory fails them. As always, remember to take care of yourself. Those memory boxes and photo albums work when you're not there. Maybe they can free you up so another caregiver can watch your person while you have lunch with a friend or see a movie.

6

Light for Dementia

No one lights a lamp to hide it behind the door: the purpose of light is to create more light, to open people's eyes, to reveal the marvels around.

—*Paulo Coelho*

My husband Joe loved to read the newspapers in the morning. Not only did he read them, but he was an enthusiastic clipper of articles that piqued his interest, and he always created an individualized stack for me. Although his ability to read was in decline, Joe still enjoyed the process of perusing and clipping.

On a cloudy day, I noticed he had skipped his favorite activity, and he seemed restless and agitated. Worried that dementia had taken another pleasure from him, I looked at his reading corner and noticed it was dark and somewhat dreary. The table, chair, and tools of his craft faded into the room's corner.

With hope, I moved his table to the window and added a reading lamp, thereby increasing the light levels. I put his paper on the table along with his cup of coffee. I laughed when he immediately gravitated to his light-filled reading corner. I hadn't even needed to suggest that he might want to read the paper.

The additional lighting for Joe's reading task not only helped him see the words on the page more clearly, but it also created a focal point that drew him in. This is because light can be empowering and stimulating for the eye's energy sensors, which can enhance perception. The bright area in Joe's field of vision likely attracted and energized his eyes, making it easier for him to focus and engage with his reading material. Overall, the increased lighting in Joe's reading corner had a positive impact on his ability to read and concentrate.

My grandmother Clara had a harrowing experience with light-induced glare one evening. While I visited for dinner, she became agitated and fearful, believing that people were spying on us and that we were in danger. She pointed to one of the caretakers and claimed that they were writing down everything we did and ate in order to first fatten us up and then take us away. As I looked out the window, I could see the glare from the bright room reflecting off the glass and creating distorted images. It was clear that Clara was seeing these reflections as people outside the window, and she was terrified.

I struggled to find a way to calm her and reassure her that we were safe. I turned to her and gave her a big smile and explained that we were seeing reflections from the room's lights. She pulled away from me and sobbed, huddling in the chair. She could not to be consoled until we returned to her room with the drapery drawn over the window.

The care facility where my grandmother lived was situated on a stunning wooded property, with a dining room that was filled with windows and flooded with natural light during the day. However, at night, the bare windows became a source of glare that distorted the reflections of people, light fixtures, and movement. This caused my grandmother and other residents with dementia to see a distorted view *filled with terrifying lights, strange people, and wild animals. After this incident, I spoke with the facility about the issue, and they installed draperies to eliminate the problem. The dining room is now a beautiful, calming space for all the residents during the day and night.*

SEEING THE WORLD

Light is a vital element in our daily lives, playing a crucial role in how we perceive and interact with the world around us. In addition to providing visual clarity, light also has the power to regulate hormones, promote sleep, and even evoke emotional responses. However, for our people with dementia, lighting can present unique challenges. Dementia can impair the brain's ability to process visual information, leading to compromised visual acuity. This can cause anxiety and difficulties in distinguishing features and obstacles, making it all the more important to carefully consider the lighting in environments. While natural light from the sun supports human health and vision, we spend the majority of our time indoors, where artificial light sources become increasingly important. In chapter 7, we will delve further into the relationship between light and color, exploring how they work together to shape our understanding and experience of the world.

Human Biology and Light

The human body has an internal clock known as the *circadian rhythm*, which helps regulate various bodily functions and activities over a twenty-four-hour period. (See figure 6.1.) The hypothalamus of the brain holds the body's clock, which is controlled by a group of nerve cells called the suprachiasmatic nucleus (SCN). The SCN receives information about incoming light from the optic nerve and sends signals to the brain to regulate alertness. As the amount of light decreases in the evening, the SCN sends signals to the body to relax.

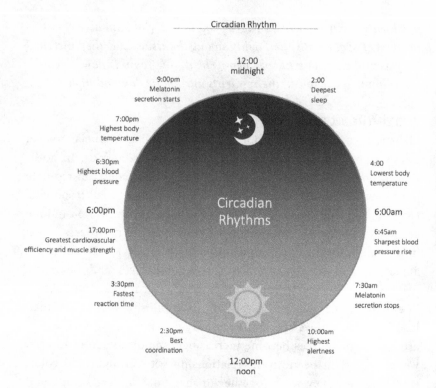

Circadian Rhythm

12:00
midnight

9:00pm
Melatonin
secretion starts

2:00
Deepest
sleep

7:00pm
Highest body
temperature

6:30pm
Highest blood
pressure

4:00
Lowest body
temperature

6:00pm

Circadian
Rhythms

6:00am

17:00pm
Greatest cardiovascular
efficiency and muscle strength

6:45am
Sharpest blood
pressure rise

3:30pm
Fastest
reaction time

7:30am
Melatonin
secretion stops

2:30pm
Best
coordination

10:00am
Highest
alertness

12:00pm
noon

FIGURE 6.1. MAP OF SOME PHYSIOLOGICAL PROCESSES ASSOCIATED WITH LIGHT-DRIVEN CIRCADIAN RHYTHMS
Natural light cycles drive our circadian rhythms. Disrupting our circadian rhythms, even in people without dementia, may lead to cognitive and behavioral issues like diminished focus, vigilance, attention, motor skills, and memory. These symptoms can subsequently result in workplace errors, reduced efficiency, or even accidents. Disrupting the circadian rhythms in people with dementia can compound the symptoms of the disease. *Source:* Illustrated by Grace Boateng.

Circadian rhythms are important for maintaining a healthy sleep-wake cycle and can be disrupted by various factors, including age and dementia.[1] Disturbances in the circadian cycle affect 25 to 60 percent of people with dementia,[2] causing sleep problems such as insomnia, sleep fragmentation,[3] and sundowning.[4] People with dementia require access to natural sunlight during the day to help synchronize their body clock and promote healthy sleep patterns.[5]

Full-spectrum light, which is light that spans the full spectrum of colors from infrared to ultraviolet, can also be beneficial for maintaining a healthy body clock. Full-spectrum light can improve visual acuity and has organic benefits related to biological processes, such as managing pigments and hormones.

Sunlight, also known as natural light or daylight, is the light emitted by the sun. It is composed of the full spectrum of colors, including infrared, visible, and ultraviolet light. Sunlight has numerous benefits for health and well-being. It helps regulate hormones, promotes healthy sleep patterns, and can increase energy levels. Many people prefer natural sunlight to artificial light, as it is important for maintaining the body's natural wake-sleep cycle. In the elderly, a lack of access to natural daylight can lead to disruptive behavior, sundowning, and a range of health problems.[6]

Artificial lighting is a manufactured source of electrical light that is designed to mimic the brightness and color of sunlight. It typically consists of a light bulb and a lamp fixture that houses the bulb. The way in which the fixtures are manipulated, the height at which they are mounted, the type of bulb used, and the variety of shielding used all contribute to the different lighting effects that can be achieved. Both natural and artificial light can be used to support your person with dementia.

The Function of Light

Light plays a vital role in the lives of people with dementia, influencing their ability to interpret the world. Light can solve problems by reducing glare, highlighting desired features, or blending objects into the background. Light can also facilitate navigation, allowing your person to walk safely down stairs. You as a caregiver will make a range of decisions related to lighting, and by understanding the characteristics of lighting—brightness, contrast, and color—you can support your person better, reduce unwanted behavior caused by a misinterpretation of the world, and provide safety.

Brightness: Brightness is an attribute of visual perception in which a source appears to be radiating light. Visual acuity issues related to dementia and aging require higher light levels than are typically found in the home.[7] Even without dementia, you need brighter light to see as you age. You can alter brightness with light bulbs, and wattage will tell you how bright a light is. For most rooms, a 60-watt bulb is standard, but your person with dementia needs a 20 percent brighter light. This means that you can replace 60-watt bulbs with 75- or 100-watt bulbs. You could also increase the number of lamps in a room.

Glare: As you increase brightness, you might cause glare. Glare is defined as the loss of visual performance produced by an intensity of light in the visual field greater than the intensity of light to which the eyes are adapted. Simply put, glare occurs when too much light enters your eye and interferes with your eye's ability to manage it. This can be a particular problem for people with dementia because their damaged brain can't always interpret the surface with glare. For instance, glare on a hard-surface floor might be interpreted as a puddle of water. This means that glare might limit mobility, contribute to falls, and cause fear or confusion. (See figure 6.2.) Causing fear or confusion in your person may generate unwanted behaviors. To support your person by reducing glare, consider the following tips:

1. Adjust the direction of your light sources: Try to aim your light sources away from your person with dementia, as glare can be especially bothersome for them. This might mean repositioning lamps or installing shades or filters on windows.
2. Use dimmer switches: Dimming the lights can help reduce glare and create a softer, more soothing atmosphere. Dimmer switches are an easy and cost-effective way to control the intensity of your lighting.
3. Choose the right bulbs: Consider using bulbs with a lower color temperature, as they tend to produce less glare. Warm white bulbs (2700K to 3000K) are a good option, and this information is available on the label.

4. Use indirect lighting: Indirect lighting, such as wall sconces or up-lights, can help reduce glare by illuminating surfaces rather than shining directly into the eyes.
5. Avoid reflective surfaces: Shiny or reflective surfaces, such as gloss paint or mirrored surfaces, can create additional glare. Try to mini-mize or eliminate these surfaces in your person's environment.

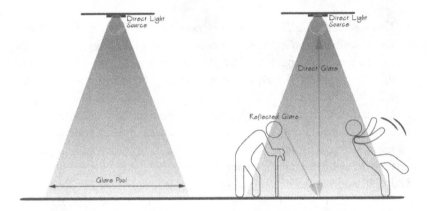

FIGURE 6.2. GLARE AND FALLS
As shown in this figure, direct lighting can form a pool of light that poses a haz-ard for people, especially people with dementia. See the list above for potential solutions. *Source:* Illustrated by Grace Boateng.

You may not realize the impact of glare on your loved one with dementia, but to them, those light patterns from the ceiling fan can be confusing and even frightening. To reduce glare and improve their experience, consider going on a glare-hunt: search for and shield any bulbs or light sources that are causing problems; reposition lamps and objects that intercept light; minimize or eliminate shiny surfaces; in-crease background light levels to create a more balanced environment; and use shades or curtains to reduce glare during peak brightness or shut windows completely at night. If you listen to your person when they express concern about something you can't see, you might find the heart of the problem lies in glare.

Contrast: Contrast, or the difference in lightness or darkness between one area and another, is important for improving visual acuity. By defining edges and surfaces, high contrast can help people identify doors against walls and highlight tripping hazards. By reducing contrast, you can help blend objects into the background.

Here are some tips for using contrast to support your person:

1. Increase contrast: To help your person identify objects and surfaces more easily, try to increase the contrast between different elements in the environment. For example, you can use light-colored walls and dark-colored doors, or place a nonslip brightly colored rug on a darker floor.
2. Use lighting to your advantage: Adjust the lighting in a room to create contrast and highlight important features. For example, you can use spotlights to highlight tripping hazards, or place a lamp near a favorite chair to make it easier to find.
3. Reduce contrast when necessary: In some cases, it may be helpful to reduce contrast to blend objects into the background. For example, you might paint a door to the basement with the same color as the wall to reduce the probability that your person will find and use that door.

Color: Color is also an important factor in lighting, with natural sunlight providing a full spectrum of colors. Manufactured light sources, such as light bulbs, vary in their ability to reproduce the full spectrum of colors. Color temperature, measured in degrees Kelvin, refers to the hue of the light and can range from warm white (2700K to 3000K) to cool white (3000K to 4100K) to daylight (5000K). To best support your person, aim for warm white light and avoid cool white. When shopping for bulbs, you can find this information on their labels.

Choosing the Right Light Bulbs for Your Person with Dementia

When it comes to choosing a light bulb for your person, there are a few key things to consider. Incandescent, fluorescent, and LED bulbs are the most common types of lighting for homes, each with their own unique benefits and drawbacks. Here is a summary of the pros and cons of each type of bulb:

Incandescent bulbs: These bulbs use a heated filament to produce light and are often preferred for their warm white color, which is closest to the full spectrum of colors. They are available in a range of brightness levels or "watts" and don't require a ballast to operate. However, they are less efficient and more expensive than fluorescent and LED bulbs, and they don't last as long due to the heat they produce.

Fluorescent bulbs: These low-pressure gas discharge lamps are known for their energy efficiency and cost-effectiveness, but they can be harsh on the eyes and cause symptoms like dryness, bloodshot eyes, headaches, vertigo, nausea, and eye pain. Fluorescent bulbs also flicker at a rapid rate, which can be especially problematic for people with dementia and the elderly. The color of fluorescent bulbs can also change over time, becoming greenish, gray, or yellow, which can be jarring for people with dementia. To minimize these issues, it is important to regularly replace fluorescent bulbs and shield the bare bulbs from view. In severe cases, special glasses that filter out the pulsing light waves can help alleviate light sensitivity from fluorescent light.

LED bulbs: These semiconductor devices use less energy, produce less heat, and last longer than incandescent bulbs, but they are more expensive to purchase. LED bulbs also produce a bluer spectrum of light, which can disrupt the circadian rhythm, and they can cause low light sensitivity in some people, similar to fluorescent bulbs.

When choosing a light bulb for a loved one with dementia, it is important to consider the impact of the light on their overall well-being. Betsy Brawley, the author of *Designing for Alzheimer's Disease*,[8] advises avoiding "cool-white" fluorescent lamps, as they are known as "cruel-white" because they are deficient in both the red and blue-violet areas of the lighting spectrum and can give skin a lifeless pallor. Instead, look for bulbs that produce a warm white light and minimize flickering and color changes to create a comfortable and soothing environment.

Lighting Applications

Good lighting is essential for people with dementia, as it can help improve visibility, reduce glare, and create a comfortable and safe environment. It can also help minimize disruptive behaviors. Here are some tips for choosing the right lighting for different areas of the home:

General illumination: In social areas like living rooms, dining rooms, and bedrooms, you might want to aim for a uniform, balanced, and comfortable level of background lighting. You can achieve this with a variety of fixtures, such as shielded downlights, table lamps, chandeliers, and sconces, placed around the room in an even pattern. Indirect lighting, which bounces off surfaces like the ceiling and walls rather than shining directly on objects or people, can create a softer, more even illumination and minimize glare. You might want to avoid direct, focused overhead lighting, as it can create shadows.

Task lighting: To support specific tasks like reading, hobbies, or grooming, you might want to provide focused lighting that can be easily positioned and adjusted. In the kitchen, for example, LED under-cabinet lights can increase brightness on work surfaces and reduce the risk of accidents. In the bathroom, sconce lighting on both sides of the mirror can help avoid shadows, and a dimmer switch can allow for adjustable light levels. You might also consider shielding light sources and using motion-sensor nightlights to ensure safety during nighttime visits to the bathroom.

Stairs: Stairs are a high-risk area for falls, especially for people with dementia, so it is important to provide well-lit pathways. Motion sensors can help ensure that lights are turned on and off as needed, and additional lighting at the top and bottom landings along the stairway can help improve visibility. LED stair lights on the treads can also provide direct lighting for each step.

Light control: Switches, sensors, dimmers, and remote controls can provide seamless control of lighting sources and their functions. Room sensors, timers, and dimmers can help adjust lighting levels to suit the needs and activities of the person with dementia. Remote controls can be useful for caregivers to manage lighting from a distance, but it is important to keep track of these small devices to prevent them from getting misplaced. Switches and controls should be easy to identify and use, and placed in view at the entrance to each room. For table lamps, it is best to have switches located near the lamp base or shade rather than on the wall, as this can be easier for the person with dementia to understand. However, some older adults may prefer mechanical switches that they are familiar with.

Emotional Lighting

Light has a powerful effect on our emotions and behaviors. Like a cat drawn to a sunbeam, people are naturally attracted to light. It brings us pleasure and awes us with beautiful sunrises, sunsets, stars, and fireflies. Even artificial light can bring delight, such as with fireworks, light shows, and technology.

Light stimulates the release of neurotransmitters called serotonin and endorphins, which produce a feeling of pleasure and well-being. These chemicals also regulate mood, motivation, appetite, and sleep, and are activated in the brain by natural sunlight.[9]

Lighting also contributes to the feeling of a space. Warm light can make a place feel welcoming, while colorful light can make it feel more festive. Light can intensify both positive and negative emotions and can improve mood and energy levels, increase appetite, and make one feel happier.[10]

Mood lighting, in particular, can help a person maintain mobility and remain more active. An example of this is the Snoezelen room, a controlled multisensory environment developed in the 1970s to mitigate anxiety. These rooms combine soft, warm lighting and quiet music with rich textures to calm anxiety and agitation.[11]

The direction of light also impacts how people feel. For example, lighting at the ceiling level can project a feeling of restraint, while light below eye level evokes individuality. To create a sense of spaciousness, use bright light on the walls and ceiling. For intimacy, use low light levels at the focal point and less light on the perimeter.

Behavioral Lighting

Lighting can have a significant impact on the behavior of people with dementia. For example, bright or flickering light can trigger negative behaviors, such as wandering or agitation, while low light can lead to depression, confusion, and behavioral issues.[12] Because light impacts people with dementia in specific ways, it can be used as an intervention to modify behaviors.

Bright light therapy: Bright light therapy (BLT) is a treatment that involves exposing an individual to intense broad-spectrum light in order to regulate the body's production of neurotransmitters like serotonin and melatonin. These neurotransmitters are involved in mood regulation and sleep patterns, and imbalances in their production can lead to conditions like depression, anxiety, and insomnia.

Bright light therapy has been studied as a potential treatment for various symptoms in individuals with dementia, including agitation, mood disturbances, and sleep problems. One study found that BLT was effective in reducing agitation in individuals with dementia who were living in a long-term care facility.[13] Another study found that BLT was effective in improving sleep quality and reducing the frequency of nighttime waking in individuals with dementia living in a nursing home.[14] A third study suggests that BLT provides immediate positive effects on mood, stimulation levels, and physiological parameters.[15]

BLT typically involves sitting in front of a specialized light therapy lamp for twenty to thirty minutes per day, either first thing in the morning or in the early evening. These lamps are available at lighting stores and on Amazon. The lamp emits light that is similar in intensity to natural sunlight, and exposure to this light can help regulate the body's production of melatonin and serotonin.

BLT is generally considered to be safe and effective, although it is important to follow the recommended guidelines for use and to consult with a healthcare provider before starting treatment. Some people may experience side effects like eye strain or fatigue while using BLT, and it is not recommended for individuals with certain eye conditions.

Tunable white light therapy: Tunable white light therapy is a treatment that involves using light sources that can be adjusted to different color temperatures in real time, synchronized with the body's circadian clock. The goal of tunable white light therapy is to regulate the body's production of neurotransmitters like serotonin and melatonin, which can help improve mood and sleep patterns.

The body's circadian clock is a natural, internal system that regulates various physiological processes, including sleep-wake cycles, hormone production, and metabolism. The circadian clock is influenced by various environmental cues, including light and temperature. Tunable white light therapy seeks to mimic these natural cues by using light sources that can be adjusted to different color temperatures throughout the day, in order to regulate the body's production of neurotransmitters and improve sleep and mood.

Tunable white light therapy is typically administered using specialized light fixtures or portable lamps that can be adjusted to different color temperatures. The individual may be exposed to the light for a set period of time each day, typically in the morning or evening. The specific protocols for tunable white light therapy may vary depending on the individual's needs and the specific treatment goals.

Tunable white light therapy has been studied as a potential treatment for various symptoms in individuals with dementia, including agitation, mood disturbances, and sleep problems. One study found that tunable white light therapy was effective in reducing agitation and improving sleep quality in individuals with dementia living in a long-term care facility.[16] Another study found that tunable white light therapy was effective in reducing the frequency of nighttime waking and improving sleep quality in individuals with dementia who live in a nursing home.[17] It is important to consult with a healthcare provider before starting tunable white light therapy.

A last piece of advice about light therapy: While the science surrounding the use of light therapies in support of people with dementia isn't settled, there are easy things you can do that will do no harm. You can let your person bask in full-spectrum light during the first two hours in the morning, and you can expose them to warm violet-colored light in the late afternoon, which will promote evening drowsiness. Preprogrammed bulbs are available on the internet that simulate sunrise and sunset wavelengths, and some even come with natural sounds.

You can promote good sleep habits by increasing fluids throughout the day and limiting them in the evening. You may want to avoid caffeine and other stimulants from late afternoon onwards. If you can keep your person active during the day, establish routines, and make wake-up and bedtime the same each day, you might also find that sleep is easier for them. Also, if you eliminate outside light at night through the use of draperies, you will both reduce potentially confusing glare and let your person's body know that nighttime is here. You might also consider an adjustment to your person's napping regime. Try to keep the naps confined to chairs, rather than beds, to encourage a lighter sleep, and try to have naps occur at the same time each day. This supports hormone production.

CONCLUSION

Lighting can clearly impact safety, but it can also impact happiness and support emotional well-being because of its role in hormone production. By considering brightness, glare, contrast, and color, you can guide your person toward—and away from—doors and stairs. By considering color and the timing of particular exposures, you can promote easier sleep patterns. Light is an attraction that draws us in with its pleasure, energy, delight, and emotion. The technology of light is ever-changing and offers solutions to enhance our lives.

7

The Language of Color

My mother, Maxcine, was a brilliant artist who had a deep love for color. Throughout her career, she explored various media, including watercolors, oil paintings, ceramics, and china painting, always using color to bring her creations to life. Then Parkinson's stripped her talents. First, tremors took her paintbrush, and then dementia robbed her of language. She could no longer tell me that the bird she painted was red or the color of her favorite dress. However, she would whirl around in that dress, commenting on the beauty of flowers. Pointing to the Christmas tree, she once said, "Oh, what beautiful candy!" Even as dementia robbed her of her words and abilities, it couldn't take away the emotions she had tied to the things she loved.

Color could confuse her. While preparing dinner after a trip to the grocery store, I couldn't find the butter, although I was pretty sure we had bought it. Mom had helped put away the groceries, and when I asked, she told me she had put the butter in the icebox. When I told her I couldn't find it, she went into the living room, opened a tall, white china cabinet and pulled out the butter. Noticing she'd placed a cucumber onto a plate,

I began to see how color defined the reality of objects for her. The white cabinet looked like a refrigerator to her even though there was no other food in it, nor was it cold. Artificial fruit was also a problem. She reached for one of her shiny, red display apples, took a big bite, and then threw it on the floor, complaining that it had no flavor and tasted awful. I began to see how color and shape defined the reality of objects for her.

Knowing how color could confuse her, we figured it could clarify too. We therefore helped redefine her world using color. To help her identify the bathroom as such, we added fluffy towels in a color she loved and would draw her eye—lavender. To help her find the white toilet, we painted the bathroom wall behind it a rich tone of eggplant. We also replaced the fake fruit with fresh fruit. However, we did continue to look for produce in the dining room cabinet. I wonder: What would have happened if we had changed its color?

COLOR AS A FORM OF COMMUNICATION

Color, defined as the visual perceptual property derived from the spectrum of light interacting with the photoreceptor cells of the eyes, can facilitate nonverbal communication, even in our infancy. As babies learn a language, they define it by shape and color: the blue car and the black cat. Babies can also learn that the red ball is for playing and the yellow duck is for bath time. These early visceral relationships with color stay with us throughout our lives.[1]

Georgia O'Keefe understood the powerful role that color can play in communication and expression. She said, "I found I could say things with color and shapes that I couldn't say any other way." As a form of nonverbal communication, color can influence our emotions, behaviors, and perceptions in powerful ways. Different colors are associated with different meanings and can convey different messages. For example, red is often associated with passion, love, and danger, while blue is often associated with calmness, trust, and dependability. Our love for color, shapes, patterns, and textures is also deeply rooted in our history as humans. Our ancestors used these aesthetic elements to understand

and navigate their environment, and as a result, we are naturally drawn to them as a source of joy and vitality. In contrast, bleak and gray colors can communicate a sense of dread and death, and our brains are hardwired to avoid such negative associations. Ultimately, the vibrant hues of color bring us a sense of life and energy, reminding us of the beauty and balance in the world around us.

Color psychology—the study of how color influences human behavior and perception—examines the ways in which color can affect our emotions, thoughts, and behaviors. For example, in marketing, using bright and vibrant colors might make a product seem more exciting and appealing, while using softer, more muted colors might make a product seem more calming and soothing. Reds and yellows are often used in restaurant branding and design because they are thought to increase appetite.

Because perception of color stems from the varying spectral sensitivity of different types of cone cells in the retina to different parts of the spectrum, colors may be defined and quantified by the degree to which they stimulate these cells. However, these physical or physiological quantifications of color do not fully explain the psychophysical perception of color appearance. In short, color conveys personal meanings that can vary from person to person.

Your person with dementia may have difficulty naming colors or identifying objects based on their color, but this does not mean that color is no longer meaningful to them. In fact, color can have a powerful emotional impact and can be a source of visual stimulation for your person with dementia. Research has shown that color can be deeply tied to emotional connections and can have symbolic, visceral, and emotional effects on the viewer.[2]

The human eye is capable of perceiving millions of different colors, thanks to the rods and cones in the retina that detect light and send signals to the brain to distinguish color. However, as we age, certain factors such as dementia, cataracts, glaucoma, macular degeneration, and diabetes can diminish our ability to see color. The aging eye may also lose sensitivity to variations in contrast between objects, leading to blurred backgrounds and difficulty differentiating colors such as blues, greens, and violets. This can also affect our ability to recognize objects and perceive depth, leading to problems such as hallucinations, searching for things on the floor, or mistaking patterns in the carpet for obstacles or steps.[3]

To better understand how someone with dementia perceives color, it's important to consider the essential components of color and how they may be affected by age-related changes in the eye. For example, the thickening of the eye's lens can cause a yellowish tint and washed-out appearance, which can make it difficult to differentiate certain colors. Caregivers can simulate this effect by coating eyeglasses with Vaseline to get a sense of how the world looks to someone with an aging eye.

In this chapter, we will explore the role that color can play in enhancing the lives of our people with dementia. While your person might have difficulty naming colors or identifying objects based on their color, research has shown that color can still have a powerful emotional impact and be a source of visual stimulation. We will discuss the importance of personal meanings and associations with color, as well as strategies for using color to create a positive and supportive environment for our people.

COLOR CONTRAST

Color contrast is an effective design tool for improving visibility. Johannes Itten was one of the first to research and develop strategies for using color contrast to define environmental features for people with dementia,[4] and you as the caregiver can use this tool to help your person. Here are some ways to use color contrast:

1. Use contrasting hues of light and dark colors to make objects stand out and draw attention to key features. For example, contrast an eggplant-colored wall with a white toilet to increase understanding and visibility.

2. Create a subtle difference in saturation by contrasting two colors with different intensities, such as midnight blue and pale baby blue. For example, use subtle contrast in bedding and blankets to create a desire in your person for comfort and up-close engagement.
3. Use warm and cool colors in contrast, such as orange and blue, to create distinction. For example, use a warm color like an orange rug next to a cool shade of blue sofa to create a temperature contrast. This will help draw your person to the sofa.
4. Use complementary colors, which are opposite each other on the color wheel (e.g., violet and yellow), to create a strong contrast. For example, use a deep hue of violet complemented by a light hue of yellow for the bathroom floor and wall tiles to maximize spatial awareness.
5. Use high contrast to make a focal point. For example, use bold colors on ramps to highlight differences in grade, or contrast the light switch with the wall color to draw attention. You can also use table settings of contrasting colors to make their meaning more obvious. If you don't want to change your table or plates, consider adding a contrasting placemat set.
6. Use low contrast to make objects blend into the background. For example, paint the exit door and frame the same color as the wall to make the door appear to recede into the background to reduce elopement problems.

Color and Emotion

Color has the ability to affect mood and emotion, and this can be especially important for people with dementia. The psychology of color links emotional responses to specific colors, and hue plays a significant role in emotion. Research has shown that brighter and more saturated colors are often associated with joy, while hues of the red-yellow spectrum are often associated with fun. On the other hand, cyan-blue hues are often associated with fear. However, it is important to note that there may be individual and cultural differences in the interpretation of color and emotion.

All color parameters are likely important when processed by a nonverbal person.[5] The link between emotions and color might be a tool you can use to improve their happiness and reduce unwanted behaviors. Each hue can elicit certain behaviors in everyday activities, as described below.

White: White is a color that can be used in design to create a sense of openness and brightness, and it can feel fresh and clean. However, as the eye ages, white may appear as beige or yellowish, and it can fade into a non-color, making it difficult to define edges and boundaries. This can be frustrating for people with dementia, who may have difficulty finding anchor points and distinguishing beginnings and endpoints in all-white spaces.

White walls can create a feeling of openness and brightness, and white is often emotionally associated with cleanliness. White can be a good choice for people with dementia who may be confused or disoriented by busy patterns or complex color schemes. However, it is important to consider the potential for glare in all-white environments and to diffuse the white with mid-tone colors to reduce this risk.

Black: Black is a color that absorbs all visible light and reflects none, making it the absence of color. This achromatic color is associated with darkness, night, and deep caverns in nature. Black, brown, and gray are among the most rejected colors by Alzheimer's patients,[6] and people with dementia may avoid black areas and other dark colors, such as deep jewel tones, dark browns, and gray, as they are difficult to distinguish from black and can feel uncomfortable.

However, gray palettes can be useful in areas that need to be avoided, such as utility rooms or electrical closets, as they are less likely to attract your person. Placing a black mat in front of a door or stairs can create the perception of holes, which may discourage people with dementia from walking on them. If you don't want your person to use particular staircases, that black mat might help.

Red: The color red has been found to have an impact on people with dementia, and research has shown that it can affect various physical and psychological processes in this population. It is one of the easiest colors for people with dementia to see, and it is often second favorite in selection tests. Some of the ways in which red can affect people with dementia include:

1. Increased appetite: Red has been found to increase appetite in people with dementia, likely due to its association with food and warmth.[7] You may consider creating red accent walls in the kitchen to bring a feeling of warmth and energy, which may stimulate appetite. Red can be used in combination with other colors, such as yellow or orange, to create a vibrant and inviting kitchen space. Incorporating red kitchen tools, such as red utensils or red appliances, can add pops of color to the kitchen and create a visually appealing space. Using red plates, cups, and other tableware can create a festive and inviting atmosphere at mealtimes, which may stimulate appetite in people with dementia. This might be super effective if red contrasts with your table; otherwise, red placemats might work better.

2. Increased alertness: Some research has found that red can increase alertness and outward orientation in people with dementia, particularly when combined with bright light.[8] This means that red coats, red cell phones, and red toothbrushes might be easier for your person to find. Does your person frequently misplace particular items? Consider changing them to red versions of themselves.

3. Increased agitation: Some studies have found that red can increase agitation and combative behavior in people with dementia, particularly those with severe cognitive impairments.[9] This means that creating overly red rooms, even kitchens, might not be appropriate for your person.

4. Decreased performance on cognitive tasks: Some research has found that red can decrease performance on cognitive tasks, such as problem-solving and memory tasks, in people with dementia.[10] If your person has a nook or table where they read or craft, you might want to minimize the red there, as they may find it distracting.

Pink: Pink, which is related to red, can also be used to support the mental health of your person with dementia. The "pinking effect" refers to the calming effect that exposure to large amounts of the color pink can have on individuals. This effect is sometimes used in color therapy to reduce combative behavior, particularly in people with dementia who may be prone to agitation and aggression.

The pinking effect is thought to be related to the calming effect of the color pink on the brain and body. Some research has suggested that the color pink can reduce heart rate and blood pressure, leading to a feeling of relaxation and calmness.[11] The pinking effect is often used in conjunction with other therapeutic interventions, such as music therapy or sensory stimulation, to create a calming environment for people with dementia.

To take advantage of the pinking effect in your own home, consider the following tips:

1. Incorporate pink into the environment: Adding pink accents or using pink as a wall color can create a calming atmosphere that may help to reduce combative behavior in people with dementia. You can incorporate pink through the use of pink pillows, blankets, curtains, or other decorative items.
2. Use pink during activities: Incorporating pink into activities, such as using pink craft materials or incorporating pink foods into meals, can help to create a calming and enjoyable atmosphere for your person with dementia.
3. Use pink in personal care items: Using pink towels, washcloths, or other personal care items can create a calming and comfortable environment for your person with dementia during hygiene routines.
4. Use pink in clothing or bedding: Wearing pink or using pink bedding can create a calming and soothing environment for your person with dementia, particularly at bedtime.

Violet-purple: Violet refers to a wide variety of shades of color between blue and red. Violet comprises red-tinted and blue hues. It has the shortest wavelength and the fastest vibration, which produces a calming effect. In nature, violet and dark purple inspire richness as the fruit of the vine, such as grapes, plums, beets, eggplant, and berries, and richly hued flowers of lavenders. In nature, violet is associated with sacred places. Violet is symbolic of a flower and defined by qualities of spirituality.

Violet is a color that can have a variety of effects on people with dementia, depending on the context in which it is presented. Some potential effects of violet on people with dementia include:

1. Calmness: Violet is often associated with calmness and spirituality, and it may have a calming effect on people with dementia. Incorporating violet into the environment through the use of violet accents or violet-colored objects may create a soothing atmosphere.
2. Improved mood: Some research has suggested that violet may have a positive effect on mood, particularly in people with dementia who may be experiencing depression or anxiety.[12] Incorporating violet into activities or the environment may help to improve mood and create a more positive atmosphere.
3. Improved memory: Some research has found that violet may have a positive effect on memory, particularly when combined with other colors such as blue or green.[13] Incorporating violet into memory exercises or other activities may help to improve memory in people with dementia.

Blue: Blue is a popular choice for individuals with dementia due to its calming and serene effects. It is important to be mindful of the intensity of blue, as too much can feel icy and distant. In nature, blue is often associated with the sea and sky, and can be incorporated into a nature-based blue palette through shades of ocean waves. The aging eye may have difficulty distinguishing between shades of blue and green, so it is important to avoid using blue in dining areas or on dishware.

To incorporate blue into the environment for individuals with dementia, consider using it in quiet areas such as bedrooms. Blue can also be paired with warm colors to avoid negative emotions. The calming qualities of blue, as well as other cool colors like green, can be beneficial for individuals who are agitated or anxious. Blue is the most preferred color among the geriatric population.[14]

Green: Green is a color that is often associated with nature and has a calming and refreshing effect. It can enhance vision, stability, and endurance, making it a good choice for environments that are meant to be relaxing and calming, such as bedrooms or living rooms. However, it is important to note that green tones may be confused with blue and should not be used as destination markers.

To incorporate the calming effects of green in the environment of your person with dementia, consider bringing nature indoors with plants or nature-inspired decor, or taking your person on trips to gardens or farmers' markets. It is also worth noting that green is the third most preferred color among the geriatric population.[15]

Yellow: Yellow is a bright, warm color that is emotionally energizing and often associated with happiness. In nature, yellow is the color of sunlight, growth, and daytime, and can be found in flowers such as sunflowers and daffodils, as well as in the yolks of eggs and the feathers of canaries. However, yellow can be difficult for people with dementia to see, as it can appear unflattering in fluorescent lighting and may reflect on skin tone, giving the appearance of illness. In addition, research has shown that exposure to large amounts of yellow can lead to aggression. Caregivers should therefore minimize exposure to yellow and consider using calming and tranquil colors such as green instead. While yellow can be an effective accent color when used in small amounts, particularly when paired with purples, it is important to be mindful of its potentially negative effects on those with dementia. In general, the geriatric population tends to prefer yellow as a color.[16] However, it is important to use caution when incorporating yellow into the environment for those with dementia, as it can cause visual fatigue and may not be well suited for use in large amounts.

Orange: Orange is a warm and attractive color that is often associated with comfort and is located between yellow and red on the visible light spectrum. It is more potent than either red or yellow and has been shown to alleviate anxiety.[17] In nature, orange is often associated with sea creatures and tropical fruits and is often seen at sunrise or sunset, where it pairs well with complementary shades of blue. For people with dementia, orange can be a great color to use in activity, dining, and social areas, as it shares many of the same properties as red.[18] When incorporating orange into the environment, it is important to consider using it in a saturated form, as this can help to create a sense of warmth and comfort.

Neutral: Neutral hues are earth tones, including shades of brown, beige, taupe, and cream, that are often difficult for people with dementia to see. In nature, neutral hues come from the earth and are often found in materials such as soil, rock, wood, and straw. Basic colors such as brown, black, and gray are often rejected by those with dementia, as they can appear flat and dull and make it difficult to distinguish objects. However, neutral colors can be successful as background colors on walls and ceilings.[19] The effect of color on dementia patients also depends on its position, context, and relationship to other features in the environment. For example, isolated neutral palettes may not be effective for those with dementia, as their perception of color tends to shift and alter depending on the hues used for ceilings, walls, floors, furnishings, artwork, and lighting. It is important to consider these factors when choosing colors for an environment designed for those with dementia.

ART-MAKING

Art-making can be an effective therapeutic intervention for your person with dementia, as it can allow them to express their thoughts, feelings, and creativity in a nonverbal way. The emotional brain is directly connected to the expressive effects of color in art, allowing those with dementia to appreciate and interact with art even if they have impaired cognitive abilities.[20] Art therapy can stimulate the brain in multiple ways and may even encourage speech. It can reduce agitation, anxiety, depression, and anger and provide a sense of accomplishment and purpose.[21]

You can engage in art-making with your person in many ways, including painting, drawing, collage, sculpture, and mixed media. For example, Maxcine enjoyed taking art classes at an adult daycare center, where she was able to rekindle her painting skills through finger painting and make collages from magazine clippings and colored pasta on yarn. Adult coloring books with topics that may interest the person with dementia can also be a fun and therapeutic activity.

You can set the mood by playing music and providing a variety of materials to choose from, such as chunky crayons, paints, and clay. Encourage creativity and playfulness, and praise your person's work. Adult day centers and intergenerational art activities can also be a great way to engage in art-making.

Even if your person does not seem interested in traditional art activities, you can still incorporate art into their lives. For example, my father-in-law was not interested in art activities, but he enjoyed looking at picture books with colorful illustrations of mountains and nature. We would sit with him and discuss the pictures, and he even pointed out a mountain house where he said his mother lived. This became a regular activity for us, and we would visit the library to find new picture books of mountains and nature to share with him. As the caregiver, you know your person's interests and passions, and this can help you choose art activities that are meaningful and engaging to them.

Visual arts tours, such as those offered by specialized programs like ARTZ, can be a meaningful and enjoyable experience for both you and your person. ARTZ is a program specifically designed for people living with dementia and their care partners that offers engagement and connection with the arts. ARTZ offers tours, which are often led by trained museum docents and educators, interactive activities such as gallery tours, art-making, and musical performances that are carefully curated to stimulate memories and emotions.

For example, my father-in-law, Joe, who was not an art or museum buff, enjoyed art tours because they allowed him to reminisce about his homeland in the Carpathian Mountains. My mother, who was an artist herself, was at home with art museums and expressed her opinions on her likes and dislikes. My grandmother Clara loved village scenes and would chat about the way of life depicted in them. Joe enjoyed religious and ethnic art, especially from Italy, Egypt, and Mesopotamia. These art tours provided an opportunity for my loved ones with dementia to engage with art and color, and to connect with their memories and emotions.

If your area does not offer specialized art tours, you can still visit a museum or gallery with your person and engage in meaningful discussions about the art. Consider choosing galleries that feature art that will interest your person, and perhaps focus on a few pieces rather than trying to see everything. If you encourage your person to share their thoughts and feelings about the art, you might be able to personalize the experience by connecting it to their own life experiences. When your person becomes tired or agitated, feel free to leave. Changing the minds of people with dementia is a challenging prospect. On the way out, consider picking up some postcards of the art you saw and continuing the conversation at home.

CONCLUSION

Color is a powerful tool that can have a significant impact on the well-being and quality of life of people with dementia. It can be used to help people with dementia see and interact with everyday objects, such as finding the door or recognizing food on their plate, and can define objects with contrast. Color can also affect mood, emotions, and cognition, and can be used to create a calming or stimulating environment. It is important to consider the individual preferences and needs of the person with dementia when choosing colors, as well as the context and purpose of the space.

Art-making can also be a therapeutic and meaningful activity for people with dementia, as it allows them to express their thoughts, feelings, and creativity in a nonverbal way. Art therapy can stimulate the brain in multiple ways and may even encourage speech. It can reduce agitation, anxiety, depression, and anger and provide a sense of accomplishment and purpose.

Visual art tours can also be rewarding and enjoyable experiences for you and your person. These tours offer interactive activities such as gallery tours, art-making, and musical performances that are carefully curated to stimulate memories and emotions.

In summary, the use of color and art-making can have a positive impact on the well-being and quality of life for your person. Because you know your person well, you know their individual preferences and needs, and this allows you to provide opportunities for engagement and expression through a variety of activities and interventions. As always, remember to be kind to yourself. Try what works for you, and when things don't, try to let it go and move on to something else. When things go badly, and they will, forgive yourself.

Technology for Dementia

The human spirit must prevail over technology.

—*Albert Einstein*

When doctors first diagnosed Maxcine with Parkinson's, she managed her medications with great care. Every Sunday evening, she put each chemical jewel in a little pillbox marked "morning," "noon," and "night." She knew these meds were taming her tremors, allowing her to stay at home. But inevitably the disease progressed, and the medications became a little more complicated. Parkinson's meds demand exact timing.

At the same time, dementia took a little bite, robbing some of her ability to read calendars and clocks. She sometimes forgot her pills, and this made her frustrated with herself, frustrated with calendars and clocks, and then frustrated with the pills themselves. When we asked her about her once-cherished pillbox, she became angry. "I don't need those stupid pills. They don't work anyway."

Soon, her Parkinson's was out of control. The erratic medication schedule sent her to the hospital. Once she was back home, our entire family intervened. We devised a plan. Each of us would take a turn to call Mom. Aunts, children, and grandchildren all wanted to help; she didn't want to go to assisted living, and we wanted to support her.

For a while it worked. These calls prompted Mom to take the meds while we waited on the phone. We all had a chance to check in, and she enjoyed all the calls with family. But dementia took another small bite, and she couldn't remember why we were all calling so frequently. When we reminded her, she felt stupid. This made her annoyed with the pills, the telephone, and all of us. Each call became a battle, and it appeared that assisted living lay in her near future.

Fortunately, my sister-in-law discovered a technical intervention—an electronic pill minder, which she named "Queenie." Queenie verbally reminded her to take the pill at the appropriate time, dispensing each like a gumball. It even called her name. It would beep and keep beeping until she removed the pills, and if she ignored it, the device would call family member after family member until someone answered.

The medication management technology was a remarkable nonthreatening intervention that enabled Maxcine to live independently for at least two additional years, and it kept her relationships with her family intact and tension free.

A QUICKLY CHANGING FIELD

The use of technology to support people with dementia has grown tremendously in recent years. The fast-paced nature of this field means that new solutions are constantly being developed and implemented, with the aim of improving the quality of life for people with dementia— and their caregivers. From assistive devices that help with daily tasks to virtual reality programs that provide cognitive stimulation, a vast and diverse range of technological options exists.[1]

Dementia is a complex disease with multiple stages and diverse symptoms. Assistive technologies can help with daily tasks and enhance quality of life. In the early stages of dementia, these technologies may allow for greater independence and lengthen the time people get to stay at home. However, as the disease progresses, the number of effective technologies decreases. The mid to late stages of dementia have the greatest need for new innovations.[2]

Recent years have seen significant growth in the development of various kinds of technology to support our people with dementia. Smart home technologies, such as connected devices with automatic lighting and GPS applications for those who may get lost, can help to keep our people with dementia safe. Motion-based games and other leisure activities may provide cognitive stimulation and assist with mobility. Medication and pain management[3] technologies, such as pill reminders, can help our people manage their medication regimen.

In this chapter, I will provide an overview of the various technological solutions available to support our people with dementia—and their caregivers. I've ensured that all discussed technology is currently available for the home and available at home improvement stores, online retailers, and specialty stores that sell products for people with disabilities. Some popular sellers include Amazon, Lowes, Home Depot, and Best Buy.

The field of technology in support of our people with dementia is constantly evolving, and the technologies discussed in this chapter may already be out of date. Consider asking the young people in your life for advice before implementing these technologies. They may be happy to impress you with their skills and wisdom!

CELEBRATING THE CAREGIVER

Caregivers of people with dementia have often been at the forefront of developing innovative solutions to address the challenges of caring for a loved one with dementia. These "workarounds" are often born out of necessity and can range from simple adaptations and existing technologies to more complex homegrown solutions.

One example of a workaround is the use of a simple tablet device with a customized home screen and large buttons, which can make it easier for a person with dementia to access information and communicate with their caregiver. Another example is the use of wearable technology, such as a GPS tracking device, to help caregivers locate a person with dementia who has wandered or is lost.

In some cases, these workarounds have inspired the development of new technologies specifically tailored to the needs of people with dementia and their caregivers. For example, the success of wearable tracking devices led to the development of more sophisticated smartwatches and other wearable technologies that offer a range of features, including fall detection, medication reminders, and emergency alert systems.

The ingenuity and resourcefulness of caregivers has been a driving force in the development of new technologies to support people with dementia, and continues to be an important source of inspiration for researchers and developers in the field. It may be that on your journey, you will discover the next important technological advance!

TECHNOLOGY THROUGH DEMENTIA'S PHASES

Dementia is a progressive disease that affects everyone differently, with symptoms ranging from the mild to the severe over the course of the disease. While the course of the disease may differ from person to person, it typically progresses through three distinct phases: early, middle, and late. The appropriate technology for each phase will vary, and it's important to be open and patient with your approach to technology, as what works in one phase may not necessarily work in another.

In the early phase, your person may still be able to live independently but may be experiencing memory lapses and difficulty with organization and planning. Assistive technology such as smartphones and smart devices, messaging, and medication management can be helpful in maintaining independence at this stage. These and other relevant technologies are described in this chapter.

Caregivers often find the middle phase most challenging since our people require the most significant care in this phase. Symptoms during this phase may include difficulty with routine tasks, changes in personality and behavior, and a decline in mobility and vision. Technology that supports daily assistance such as adaptive clothing and message management may be useful during this stage. However, technology for the middle phase is still lacking and more is needed to support activities involving daily living, confusion, personal hygiene issues, and sleep problems, which are some of the most challenging symptoms.

In the late phase or final stage of the disease, the person with dementia will be completely reliant on caregivers for support. Symptoms during this stage may include a loss of mobility and compromised communication, as well as an increased risk of infections and pneumonia. As cognition declines, pain interpretation becomes more challenging.[4] Technology that focuses on comfort, dignity, and pain management can be beneficial during this stage. The sections below describe technologies that you might find useful through the various phases.

TECHNOLOGIES IN SUPPORT OF PEOPLE WITH DEMENTIA

Technologies that promote safety, daily living, and entertainment can have a positive impact on the autonomy and independence of people with dementia, as well as help to manage potential safety risks. Equally important, they can reduce your worry and your stress, making caregiving easier and sometimes more fun. In this section, I will discuss each of those categories.

Technology for Safety

Having dementia increases risks in so many categories: falling, getting lost, burns, accidental poisonings, mis-medicating, and many others. Worrying about your person adds another risk—risk to your physical and mental health. Assistive technologies can make dementia care a little more manageable and a little less stressful. I discuss some available technologies to improve safety here. You might think of some of your own!

Monitoring systems: Smart home monitoring systems often use a combination of sensors, cameras, and other smart devices to monitor the home environment and send alerts to caregivers in real time. These systems can be integrated with a wide range of devices, including smart thermostats, smoke detectors, door and window sensors, and more.[5]

Caregivers can find a variety of home monitoring systems to help their person manage potential safety risks and to promote independence. Here are some examples:

1. Smart door and window sensors: These sensors can alert caregivers if your person opens a door or window, which can be helpful for ensuring their safety and preventing them from wandering outside.
2. Smart motion sensors: These sensors can detect movement in the home and send an alert to you if your person has not been active for an extended period of time.
3. Smart smoke and carbon monoxide detectors: These detectors can alert caregivers if there is a fire or gas leak in the home.
4. Smart bed and chair sensors: These sensors can detect when your person gets in or out of bed or a chair and send an alert to caregivers if your person has not been active for an extended period of time.
5. Smart medication dispensers: These dispensers can dispense medication at scheduled times and send reminders to your person.

There are many other types of systems available, each with its own set of features and benefits. You may even invent your own.

Safe kitchens: The kitchen is a high-risk area for accidents for people with dementia, as their memory loss may cause them to forget how to use appliances and potentially put them in danger. To make the kitchen safer, there are several technological solutions that can be employed.

One solution is the use of device-monitoring systems that alert caregivers if the stove is turned off or left unattended. These are called cooktop safety sensors. Motion detectors can also be helpful in preventing accidents. For example, if a person with dementia is cooking and steps out of view of the motion detector for more than five minutes, the device can put the stove into standby mode and stop the cooking process. Shut-off timers that work in conjunction with motion sensors can also be useful in detecting when a stove has been left unattended. For example, the iGuardStove Plug-in Electric Range Monitor automatically shuts off your stove after fifteen minutes with no activity near it, preventing unattended stove fires before they can start. As of the writing of this book, this technology is expensive, but it may make sense for you anyway.

Other technologies such as stove top covers and locking knobs can also help to reduce the risk of accidents in the kitchen. If your stove has a gas pilot light, you may consider replacing it with an electric starter. You may also want to keep electric appliances tucked away off the counter, with cords disconnected.

In the sink area, you can install an automatic turn-off on the faucet and disguise or disconnect garbage disposal switches. You may also consider turning down the hot water settings and using alternative cooking methods, such as the microwave, as well as electric tea kettles and coffee pots with automatic shutoffs. These measures can help to minimize the use of the stove and reduce the risk of accidents in the kitchen. They may reduce your own worry and also allow your person to live at home longer.

Motion sensor lights: Motion sensor lights can be a useful tool for increasing safety and independence in the home. Movement activates these lights, and you can easily install them in various locations throughout your home.

For instance, you might consider installing motion sensor lights on the stairs. Navigating stairs can be a difficult and potentially dangerous task. Additionally, lighting might make them more navigable, even if your person doesn't think of it themself.

You might consider adding motion sensor lights in the bathroom. Your person might feel disoriented and confused when getting up to use the bathroom during the night. Motion sensor lights can help guide your person to the toilet, thereby reducing the risk of accidents.

Last, you might consider adding motion sensor lights to the kitchen. For people with dementia, cooking can be a difficult and potentially dangerous task. By installing motion sensor lights in the kitchen, your person will have the benefit of additional illumination as they navigate around the kitchen, potentially reducing the risk of accidents and injuries.

Motion sensor lights for people with dementia are available in many places. You can find them at home improvement stores, online retailers, and specialty stores that sell products for people with disabilities. Some popular options include Amazon, Lowes, Home Depot, and Best Buy. You can also check with local lighting stores or electricians to see if they have any recommendations or can install the lights for you, although some can be placed using adhesive tape and run on batteries, making them super easy for anyone to install. With a little research, you can compare prices and features before making a purchase.

Smart locks: Smart locks are a type of lock that is easy for caregivers to use but difficult for people with dementia to manipulate. These locks do not require keys and may not even look like traditional locks, making them a good option for preventing access to potentially hazardous areas such as basements, garages, and cabinets with dangerous items. These locks are easy to install and widely available, making them a convenient and effective way to keep your person safe. For a low-tech solution, baby locks may also work.

My mom had dementia before smart locks were commonly available. Worried she might fall down the stairs, I installed a padlock on the door. Undaunted, she pulled a screwdriver out of the junk drawer and removed the entire mechanism. A smart lock might have solved this problem—or it might have inspired her to find a hacksaw. I wonder what would have happened if I had painted the door and its frame to match the surrounding wall.

Tracking technology: One common risk for our people with dementia is the possibility of getting lost and confused to the degree that they can't ask for help. To help prevent this, caregivers can use wearable GPS tracking devices that can locate a wandering loved one and provide peace of mind. These devices can be worn on the body or inserted into shoes, and can alert caregivers if their loved one leaves a specific area. Some versions even have the capability to alert emergency personnel to ensure a safe and speedy recovery. These are easily available and come with apps for your smartphone.

Medical monitoring: Medical monitoring technology can be an important resource for caregivers of people with dementia, helping to ensure that their loved one receives the medical care and attention they need.

One type of medical monitoring technology is wearable devices, such as smartwatches or other wearable sensors. These devices can track a person's vital signs, such as heart rate and blood pressure, and alert caregivers to any changes that may indicate a potential health problem. Wearable devices may also include features such as fall detection, which can alert caregivers if their loved one has taken a fall and may need assistance.

Another type of medical monitoring technology is remote monitoring systems, which allow caregivers to remotely monitor their loved one's health using sensors or other devices placed in the home. These systems may include sensors that track a person's vital signs, as well as devices such as smart pillboxes that alert caregivers if a person has not taken their medication as prescribed. Remote monitoring systems may also include video surveillance, allowing caregivers to remotely check in on their loved one and ensure that they are receiving the care they need.

Pill management: Pill management technology refers to devices and systems that are used to help people with dementia remember to take their medication as prescribed. These technologies can range from simple pill organizers or reminder devices to more complex systems that are connected to a person's healthcare provider and can dispense medication automatically.

One example of pill management technology is the use of pill organizers, which are containers that are divided into compartments for each day of the week. The compartments are labeled with the time of day, and the person with dementia can fill each compartment with the correct medication for that time. This can help to ensure that the person is taking the correct dosage at the correct time.

Another example of pill management technology is the use of reminder devices, which can be set to alert the person with dementia when it is time to take their medication. These devices can take the form of an alarm on a smartphone or a wearable device, such as a smartwatch or a bracelet.

More advanced pill management systems may use automation to dispense medication at the correct time. These systems can be connected to a person's healthcare provider and can be programmed to dispense the correct dosage of medication at the appropriate intervals. Some of these systems may also have features such as automatic refill reminders and the ability to alert a caregiver if the person misses a dose. Queenie in the opening story is one such device.

Car safety: Taking the keys away from a person with dementia can be a challenging and emotional task for caregivers. It is important to be aware of their driving skills, as they may be able to continue driving for a few years after their diagnosis in the early stages of dementia. However, it is ultimately the caregiver's responsibility to ensure that their person is not a danger on the road.

There are several warning signs to watch out for, such as difficulty finding the windshield wipers, confusion about how to use the car's controls, getting lost easily, and failing to obey traffic laws. If you are concerned about your person's driving abilities, you can have them take a driving test or obtain a doctor's letter stating that they are no longer fit to drive. However, even with these documents, it may be difficult to convince your person to give up their car. My late husband and I agreed that he should no longer drive, but those conversations were forgotten when the need to drive was upon him. My late mom, who could no longer make a cup of tea, could ferret out keys from hidden places, start the engine, drive off—and proceed to get lost in the town where she'd spent twenty years. She did this after agreeing, time and time again, that she should not be driving.

Stopping cold turkey might be too hard for some people, both caregivers and people with dementia. One way to ease the transition is to gradually decrease their need to drive by offering alternative transportation options. You can take them to their desired destinations most of the time, thereby slowly limiting their time behind the wheel. Maybe you can have groceries and other necessities delivered, and use ride-sharing services or public transportation. With both of you driving less, your person might feel less inclined to drive. Your person may enjoy using the electric shopping carts in grocery and big-box stores, as they can bring joy and a sense of independence even in the late stages of dementia.

When the time comes to take away the keys, be firm but kind, and consider securing the keys (better than I did with my mom), hiding the car, disabling the vehicle, or even getting rid of the car. I gave away my late husband's car to someone he wanted to help. Every time he looked for his car, we had a good conversation about someone he admired. He usually forgot he wanted to drive someplace. Try to remember that driving is a privilege, not a right, and it is important to ensure that your person is not a danger to themselves or others on the road.

Technologies in Support of Daily Living

Many existing technologies that are used primarily for people without dementia have been successfully adapted to support you and your person. In this section, I discuss some of them.

Smart speakers: Smart speakers, such as Amazon's Alexa and Google's Home, are voice-activated devices that can be used to play music, set reminders, answer questions, and perform a variety of other tasks through voice commands. These devices can provide a simple and intuitive way for your person to access information and perform various tasks without the need for a computer or smartphone.

Some smart speakers also offer features specifically designed for people with dementia. For example, the Amazon Echo Show can display photos and play videos, which can be helpful if your person has difficulty understanding spoken instructions. The Echo Show also has a feature called "Drop In," which allows caregivers to call in and speak with their person through the device's built-in speaker and microphone.

In addition to providing a convenient and easy-to-use interface, smart speakers can also help promote independence and improve quality of life for people with dementia. For example, your person with dementia might use a smart speaker to play their favorite music, set reminders for medication or appointments, or get information about the weather or news.

Adapted phones: There are several ways to adapt a smartphone to make it easier to use for people with dementia:

1. Simplify the home screen: Remove unnecessary icons and widgets from the home screen, and keep only the most essential apps visible. This can reduce confusion and make it easier for the user to find the apps they need.
2. Increase the text size and contrast: Make the text on the screen larger and increase the contrast between the text and the background to make it easier to read.
3. Use a lock screen with large buttons: Consider using a lock screen with large buttons or a PIN pad, so the user can easily unlock the phone without struggling with a fingerprint or facial recognition.
4. Use a voice assistant: Enable a voice assistant like Siri or Google Assistant so the user can easily make phone calls or send messages by voice command.
5. Set up emergency contact information: Add emergency contact information to the lock screen, so it is easily accessible in case of an emergency.
6. Use a case with large buttons: Consider using a phone case with large, easy-to-press buttons, so the user can easily make phone calls or access other features without struggling with small buttons.

Video chat services: Video chat services allow for real-time communication and visual connection even when your person with dementia is unable to physically be present. Some popular video chat services include Skype, Zoom, and FaceTime. You can access these services through a computer, smartphone, or tablet, and you can hold virtual visits with family and friends, participate in social activities, and attend medical appointments.

In addition to providing a way to stay connected, video chat services might also be beneficial for maintaining cognitive stimulation and engagement. You can use video chat to interact with your person through activities such as reminiscing, playing games, or discussing current events.

You might want to set up the video chat service in a way that is user-friendly for your person, such as using large buttons and a simple interface, and provide any necessary assistance with using the technology. Consider asking the young people in your life for help and ideas. It may even promote their connection with your person.

Adaptive clothing: As the caregiver, you can adapt your person's wardrobe to support their ability to cope with dementia. Here are some ways:

1. Choose clothing with easy-to-use closures: Clothing with zippers, Velcro, or snaps can be easier for people with dementia to put on and take off compared to clothing with buttons.
2. Label clothing: It can be helpful to label clothing with tags or sew-on labels to help people with dementia identify which items go together and know which articles of clothing belong to them.
3. Choose clothing with contrasting colors: People with dementia may have difficulty distinguishing between similar colors, so choosing clothing with high contrast can help them identify which items are theirs.
4. Consider comfort: People with dementia may have sensory processing issues, so it's important to choose clothing that is comfortable to wear and avoid items that may be itchy or scratchy.

5. Avoid loose-fitting clothing: Clothing that is too loose may be difficult for people with dementia to manage, as it may get caught on
   objects or be difficult to put on properly. Overall, it's important to
   consider the individual needs and preferences of the person with
   dementia when selecting clothing.

Technology in clothing: Technology can be embedded into clothing to
support people with dementia in ways that may be helpful to you.

1. GPS tracking: Clothing with built-in GPS tracking can help caregivers keep track of their person if they wander or get lost. These tracking devices can be embedded into clothing or attached as a small,
   discreet device that can be worn on a belt, in a pocket, or in a shoe.
2. Medication reminders: Clothing with built-in medication reminders
   can help people with dementia remember to take their medication
   on time. These reminders can be in the form of vibrating alerts or
   audio prompts from watches, bracelets, or necklaces.
3. Fall detection: Clothing with built-in sensors can detect when a person with dementia has fallen and send an alert to caregivers, helping
4. to prevent serious injuries. Through fall detection and by getting
   help to the person quickly, these devices prevent complications, further injury, and even death.
5. These can look like bracelets, watches, or necklaces.

Timekeeping: Several technologies can help people with dementia
keep track of time. One option is a digital clock with large, easy-to-
read numbers. This can help people with dementia understand what
time it is, even if they are experiencing cognitive decline. They may be
simple digital clocks with large, easy-to-read numbers, or they may be
more complex devices with features such as alarms, timers, and visual
indicators for different times of day. Some dementia clocks use images
or colors to help people understand the passage of time, and others
may have features such as calendars or weather indicators. These clocks
can help people with dementia maintain their daily routines and stay

on track with medications and other important tasks. These clocks are easily purchased.

Another option is a watch with an alarm function, which can be set to remind the person to take medications or perform other tasks at specific times. Smartphone apps can also be used to set reminders and alarms, and can be customized to provide additional information such as the day of the week or the weather forecast. Additionally, calendars with large print or electronic calendars that can be accessed on a computer or smartphone can help people with dementia stay organized and remember important events or appointments.

Message management: Several technologies can help manage messages for our people with dementia. Electronic message centers, also known as reminder systems, can be programmed to play back recorded messages at specific times throughout the day. These messages can remind your person to take their medication, make appointments, or perform other tasks. Electronic message centers can also be set up to display written messages or visual reminders, such as flashing lights or colors. In addition to electronic message centers, apps available for smartphones and tablets can send reminders and alerts to caregivers or their people with dementia. These apps can be customized to send reminders at specific times or intervals, and can even be programmed to send alerts in the event of an emergency or if certain tasks are not completed. Low-tech options, such as chalkboards or dry erase boards, can also be useful for leaving written reminders in a visible location. Joe loved our chalkboard, sometimes adding to it and always commenting on the planned events for the day.

Technology for Fun

Creating fun for our people with dementia can have several benefits. It can help improve their quality of life, reduce feelings of loneliness and isolation, and increase their sense of purpose. All of this reduces stress for you, the caregiver. In addition, engaging in enjoyable activities can help your person maintain or improve their cognitive and physical abilities, and may even have the potential to slow the progression of the disease. Providing opportunities for fun and leisure can also be a way for caregivers and family members to connect with their loved ones and build positive relationships.

Different types of technology can be used to create fun for people with dementia. High-technology options include virtual reality headsets, interactive video games, and touchscreen tablets. These types of technology can provide immersive and engaging experiences that can help to stimulate the mind and provide a sense of enjoyment. I discuss some of those here.

Low-technology options for creating fun for people with dementia include simple games and puzzles, sensory toys, and creative activities such as coloring or painting. These types of activities can help to engage the senses and provide a sense of accomplishment and enjoyment.

Overall, the key to creating fun for your person is to find activities and technologies that are tailored to their interests and abilities—and yours. By providing a variety of options and regularly introducing new activities, you can help to keep things interesting and engaging for your person and yourself.

Talking photo albums: Talking photo albums are devices that allow users to record audio messages or descriptions for each photograph in the album. These devices can be helpful for people with dementia, as they may struggle with short-term memory and have difficulty remembering the details of a photograph or event. By listening to the recorded audio messages, individuals with dementia can access additional information about the photograph and better understand the context and significance of the event or person depicted in it. Talking photo albums can be a helpful tool for improving memory and communication, and may also provide a source of comfort and enjoyment for people with dementia. These are available for purchase at many online retailers, and some allow family members to add photos and voices via web browsers.

Care robots: Care robots can support our people with dementia by improving their quality of life and alleviating the burden on caregivers. Care robots are designed to provide social interaction, communication, and, sometimes, assistance with tasks such as reminding people to take their medication or providing companionship.

One well-known care robot is Paro, a baby seal robot that has been studied for its clinical effects on people with special needs for more than two decades. It is designed to provide comfort and companionship through its appearance and actions, such as making eye contact and responding to touch and voice. Paro has been found to have a positive impact on the psychological well-being of older adults, particularly in reducing depression and loneliness. However, some studies have also found that its effects may be limited and may depend on the individual and their level of cognitive impairment.

Care robots have also been used in home settings to support older adults who are living independently. In these situations, robots can provide reminders for tasks such as taking medication or providing information about appointments. They can also serve as a source of social interaction and companionship for people who may be isolated.

More affordable options, such as Joy for All cats and dogs, have also been tested in care home settings. These robot pets have been found to have a positive impact on the well-being of care home residents, including reducing neuropsychiatric symptoms and occupational disruptiveness for caregivers. Qualitative studies have also suggested that these robots are well accepted and suitable for lonely individuals, and that their use can provide entertainment and help to reduce anxiety and agitation. Joy for All and Perfect Petzzz are available for purchase online.

Virtual reality (VR): VR technology has been used in the field of dementia care to provide cognitive and sensory stimulation, as well as to facilitate social interaction and reminiscence therapy. VR experiences can range from simple virtual nature scenes to more complex interactive environments that simulate real-life situations or past experiences.

One study found that VR was effective in reducing agitated behavior and improving social interaction in people with dementia.[6] Another study found that VR reminiscence therapy was effective in improving mood and reducing depression in people with dementia.[7]

As of the writing of this book, there are specialized companies that bring VR to assisted living facilities and take people on virtual tours of destination locations. You can bring VR to your home if you have (a) the space to attach the camera sensors (think of an unused bedroom or office), (b) about $1,000 for the computer and associated gear, and (c) a grandchild to hook it all up and select the right application for your person. While your grandchild might use VR to slay brain-eating zombies, you and your person might be more comfortable using it to visit Rome.

Other big-ticket interactive gaming options: Imagine a giant koi pond on your living room floor with fish that respond to your actions. Imagine birds that fly away as you walk through Greece. Interactive projection technology, which uses sensors to detect movements and translate them into on-screen graphics and sounds, makes these possible. Some companies cater to people with dementia and offer products that can be brought into your home. For example, a company called LUMOplay makes games such as *Follow the Leader*, which involves following the movements of an on-screen character, and *Memory Match*, which challenges players to remember and replicate sequences of movements. Other games that might be suitable for people with dementia include *Musical Chairs*, which involves moving to different spots on the screen in time with music, and *Hula Hoop*, which involves moving their arms and body to keep on-screen hula hoops moving. The companies listed below make both VR and projector-based games to support people with dementia:

1. Dementia VR: This company offers a range of virtual reality experiences designed to stimulate the senses and promote relaxation for people with dementia. The content includes nature scenes, such as

waterfalls and forests, as well as cultural and historical experiences, such as visits to famous landmarks and museums.

2. LUMOplay: This company offers interactive virtual reality experiences designed to engage and entertain people with dementia. The content includes nature scenes, such as beach and mountain views, as well as interactive games and activities.

3. Reminiscence VR: This company offers virtual reality experiences designed to help people with dementia reminisce about their past and stimulate their memories. The content includes scenes and experiences from different time periods, such as the 1950s or the 1970s, as well as cultural and historical events.

Smart technology gaming: Smart technology can be used to create interactive and engaging games for people with dementia. These games can be played on devices such as smartphones, tablets, or smart TVs, and can help stimulate the mind, improve memory and cognitive function, and provide enjoyment and a sense of accomplishment.

Some examples of smart technology games for people with dementia include those listed below. The young people in your life might have some additional suggestions.

- Lumosity is a brain-training program that offers a range of games and activities designed to improve cognitive skills such as memory, attention, and problem-solving. The program is available on a variety of devices, including smartphones, tablets, and computers.
- iFish Pond is a smartphone game that involves tapping the screen to catch fish. The game is designed to improve hand-eye coordination and reaction time, and can be played by people of all ages.
- Elevate: This brain-training program offers a range of games and activities designed to improve cognitive skills such as language, math, and critical thinking.
- Peak: This brain-training program offers a variety of games and activities designed to improve cognitive skills such as memory, attention, and problem-solving.

- CogniFit: This brain-training program offers a range of games and activities designed to improve cognitive skills such as memory, attention, and executive function.

Low-tech games: Traditional low-tech games can also entertain your person, and maybe yourself. I've listed several main categories below, and most of these have been adapted to play on cell phones, computers, or tablets.

- Memory games: Memory games, such as matching cards or Concentration, can be adapted for smart technology and played on devices such as tablets.
- Word games: Word games, such as crossword puzzles or Scrabble, can be adapted for smart technology and played on devices such as smartphones or tablets.
- Physical games: Physical games, such as bowling or golf, can be adapted for smart technology and played on devices such as tablets or smart TVs. Xbox and Nintendo make games that are physical and fun for everyone.
- Puzzle games: Puzzle games, such as jigsaw puzzles or Tetris, can be played on devices such as tablets or smartphones.

Music: Music is a powerful and effective intervention for all phases of dementia. It can provide enjoyment, improve mood, and stimulate the mind. There are many different types of music technology available, including:

- Smart speakers: Smart speakers, such as Amazon's Alexa and Google's Home, can play music on demand through voice commands. These devices can be particularly useful for people with dementia, as they can provide a simple and intuitive way to access music.
- Music streaming services: Music streaming services, such as Spotify and Pandora, allow users to access a wide variety of music through their computer or smartphone. These services often have features

such as personalized playlists and radio stations, which can help people with dementia discover new music.

- Digital music players: Digital music players allow users to store and play music on the go. These devices can be helpful for people with dementia who want to listen to music while they are out and about.

This might be a fun activity to bring in the young people in your life. Our granddaughter offered a perfect solution for Joe. She sat interviewing him, playing bits of music, and then she put together the perfect playlist, just for him. She added it to his phone, which was then made available for all our devices. He enjoyed his music for months. In hospice, we added a comfortable headset and he listened to his favorite music through his last moments. Today, I still pull out his playlist and reminisce about his favorite music.

Podcasts: You may be of the age and technological experience that when you read the word *podcast* you don't know exactly what they are. A podcast is a digital audio file that is available for download onto any internet-enabled device or can be "streamed" (played "live" through/ over the internet). Podcasts are flourishing in popularity and can be accessed through streaming services like Spotify and Apple Podcast through any Wi-Fi connection in your home, coffee shop, or even doctor's waiting room (just ask the front desk!). Podcasts are typically available as a series, and new episodes are released on a regular basis. Podcasts can be downloaded and played on a variety of devices, including smartphones, tablets, and computers.

Podcasts cover a wide range of topics and genres, including news, sports, comedy, drama, music, and more. People have created podcasts that feature old-time radio shows, which may be of interest to people with dementia and provide all the benefits of reminiscence therapy. Some examples include:

1. *Radio Days*: This podcast features classic radio shows from the 1930s, 1940s, and 1950s, including old-time radio dramas, comedies, and more.
2. *Old-Time Radio Researchers* (OTRR): This podcast features a variety of old-time radio shows, including dramas, comedies, mysteries, and more.
3. *RadioClassics*: This podcast features a selection of classic radio shows, including old-time radio dramas, comedies, mysteries, and more.
4. *The Classic Radio Show*: This podcast features a variety of classic radio shows, including old-time radio dramas, comedies, mysteries, and more.

If you have never accessed a podcast, I'm here to help, although you could ask a young person in your life too. There are several ways to listen:

1. Smartphone or tablet: One of the most common ways to access podcasts is through a smartphone or tablet. There are many podcast apps available for both iOS and Android devices, such as Apple Podcasts and Google Podcasts, that allow users to discover and subscribe to podcasts. Once a podcast is downloaded, it can be played offline, making it convenient to listen to on the go.
2. Computer: Podcasts can also be accessed on a computer through a web browser. Websites such as Spotify and Apple Podcasts allow users to search for and listen to podcasts online.
3. Smart speakers: Smart speakers, such as Amazon's Alexa and Google's Home, can also be used to play podcasts. Users can ask the smart speaker to play a specific podcast or search for podcasts by topic.
4. Radio: Some podcasts are also available on the radio. Many public radio stations have programs that feature podcasts, and some podcasts are also available on satellite radio.

Television and film: Television and movies can be a valuable source of entertainment and enjoyment for you and your person. Watching television and movies can provide a sense of familiarity and comfort, and can be a helpful way to relax and unwind. If your person has a favorite movie or show, you can play it over and over again. They will not remember that they watched it only last week. My late husband would have watched *Phantom of the Opera* every night if possible.

Several options for accessing television and movies exist. These include:

1. Cable or satellite television: Traditional cable or satellite television packages offer a wide variety of channels and programming, including movies, television shows, and more.
2. Streaming services: Streaming services, such as Netflix, Hulu, and Amazon Prime, offer a wide selection of movies and television shows that can be accessed online. These services often have features such as personalized recommendations and the ability to create a watchlist and save shows for later, which can be helpful for people with dementia.
3. DVDs or Blu-rays: DVDs and Blu-rays can be a convenient way to watch movies and television shows at home. Many classic movies and television shows are available on DVD or Blu-ray, which can be a great source of nostalgia for people with dementia.

When trying to figure out what to watch, consider keeping content simple. Complex plots may lose attention. Old musicals are popular, and even if the story is lost, music can keep your person engaged. Concerts, choirs, folk groups, and dance, including ethnic dances, may also be engaging to your person. Sports are a popular genre to engage the whole family.

Several channels and services offer classic movies, which may be of interest to your person. Some examples include:

1. Turner Classic Movies (TCM): This cable and satellite television channel is dedicated to classic movies from the 1920s to the 1980s. TCM offers a wide selection of classic movies, including many that are not available on other channels or services.
2. American Movie Classics (AMC): This cable and satellite television channel offers a selection of classic movies from the 1930s to the 1980s, as well as contemporary films.
3. Criterion Channel: This streaming service offers a wide selection of classic and contemporary films, including many that are considered to be "criterion" films, or important and influential works.

Keeping your person comfortable may allow them to focus better. When using television, you might want to pay attention to some of the following:

1. Volume: It's important to set the volume at a level that is comfortable and easy for your person to hear. If the volume is too low, it may be difficult for you person to hear and follow the audio, while if the volume is too high, it may be overwhelming or confusing.
2. Closed captions: Closed captions are text versions of the audio in a television show or movie, which can be helpful for people with hearing loss or difficulty understanding spoken dialogue. Many streaming services and cable or satellite packages offer closed captions, and most television sets also have a closed captioning setting that can be turned on or off.
3. Screen definition: The screen definition, or resolution, of a television or device can affect the clarity and detail of the image. For people with vision impairments, a higher screen definition may be helpful to improve the visibility of the content. Many televisions and devices offer options to adjust the screen definition, and some streaming services also offer options to adjust the video quality.

CONCLUSION

In summary, trying new technology can be intimidating, especially when you're trying to help your person. However, embracing technology can help promote independence, manage potential safety risks, and provide peace of mind. Here are some tips for tackling new technology.

Take it slow, seek out resources and support, don't be afraid to ask for help, and be patient. It's important to take the time to understand and learn about the technology before trying to use it. Don't feel like you have to jump in and use all of the features at once. Start with the basics and work your way up to more advanced features as you become more comfortable.

There are many resources and support groups available to help you learn about and use new technology. Look for online tutorials, user manuals, or support forums that can help you understand how to use the technology. You may also be able to find local support groups or classes that can provide guidance and assistance.

If you are struggling to understand or use the technology, don't be afraid to ask for help. You can ask a friend or family member for assistance or seek out professional support if needed.

Learning and using new technology can be frustrating, and it's important to be patient and not get discouraged. Remember that it takes time to learn and adapt to new things, and it's okay to make mistakes along the way. Try to remember to be kind to yourself.

9

The Joy of Nature

Look! Look! Deep into nature, and you will understand everything.

—*Albert Einstein*

Joe, who was suffering from mid-stage dementia, was moved to a rehabilitation facility to recover from surgery and a difficult hospital stay. During his time at the facility, I would visit him daily with my small dog, Klynka. Klynka was always overjoyed to see Joe and would perform her happy dance as a greeting ritual. The presence of Klynka not only brought joy and calm to Joe but also to the other residents she encountered.

Pet therapy, or simply the presence of an animal, can provide a strong and biophilic connection. Klynka knew exactly where Joe's room was and would race toward him as soon as we arrived at the facility. Once in his room, she would jump onto his bed and snuggle up next to him. This ritual continued even after his discharge and until the day he passed away. As Joe grew more fragile, Klynka's bond with him only grew stronger. She would bring him her squeaky toy, tucking it into his hand before curling up next to him. In the end, Klynka never left his side, always offering him comfort and companionship. She was in his bed when he passed.

BIOPHILIA

The concept of *biophilia*, or the love of nature, has long been recognized as an important aspect of human well-being. From ancient sacred springs to modern-day therapy sessions in nature, humans have always sought out the calming and rejuvenating effects of the natural world. In fact, new and abundant research has shown that being in nature can have a positive impact on our physical and mental health, as well as our overall sense of well-being.

One way to understand biophilia is through the work of Edward O. Wilson, who defines it as "a deliberate attempt to translate an understanding of the inherent human affinity to affiliate with natural systems and processes."[1]

In other words, humans have a natural tendency to seek out and connect with nature, and this connection can be beneficial for our survival and well-being. This idea is further supported by the work of Stephen Kellert, who classifies biophilic attributes in terms of their human value. Kellert argues that the intrinsic value of nature is often overlooked, but is actually an important part of our subconscious drive to protect ourselves and find balance in the world.[2]

Despite the importance of nature in our lives, modern society often separates us from the natural world. Many of us spend more than 90 percent of our time indoors, surrounded by the built environment. However, nature can still be a guiding force in our lives, offering us balance and harmony even when we are not physically surrounded by it. When we watch the movements of plants in our kitchen or watch the moon rise through our windshield, that frisson of pleasure brings the benefits associated with biophilia.

Nature should be incorporated in our lives, even when housebound, to support our health and well-being. A recent review study[3] found that increased greenspace exposure was associated with improved health outcomes in several areas, including decreased stress levels, lower blood pressure and heart rate, improved cholesterol levels, and reduced risk of preterm birth, type 2 diabetes, and all-cause mortality. Neurological outcomes, cancer-related outcomes, and respiratory mortality also improved with exposure to greenspace. Another review study found that exposure to greenspace improves mental well-being, particularly life satisfaction.[4] Exposure to nature can help strengthen our sense of self, stimulate our senses and emotions, improve our awareness, and clarify our values and motivations.

Regarding dementia, studies[5] show that exposure to greenspace throughout adulthood reduces the likelihood that people will contract dementia as they age, probably because people who live near greenspace breathe cleaner air (social justice, anyone?). Another study found that living in areas with more greenspace was associated with faster thinking, better attention, and higher overall cognitive function, which translated to being 1.2 years younger from a cognitive perspective. While this too raises social justice issues since people with higher socioeconomic status tend to live in areas with more green space, this study supports the idea that green space exposure can reduce the risks of cognitive decline and dementia in older adults.[6]

Exposure to nature benefits the elderly living in assisted living facilities too. For this population, looking at greenery from windows in common areas such as lounge and dining areas has been shown to protect residents from stress and improve their quality of life. Locating residents in areas with such outdoor views may prevent their psychological condition from worsening.[7] Other researchers found that as tree cover around facilities increased, depressive symptoms decreased, regardless of the racial or socioeconomic characteristics of the residents.[8] Also, exposure to greenery, particularly garden use, improves residents' mental well-being.[9] Even having indoor plants in facilities improves mental health by reducing stress, depressive symptoms, and negative emotions.[10]

The concept of biophilia, or the love of nature, has been recognized as an important aspect of human well-being for centuries. Studies have shown that being in nature can have a positive impact on our physical and mental health, as well as our overall sense of well-being. Many of us spend a large portion of our time indoors, separated from the natural world, but nature can still be a guiding force in our lives, offering balance and harmony even when we are not physically surrounded by it. This is particularly important for older adults, including our people with dementia, as exposure to nature can help strengthen their sense of self, stimulate their senses and emotions, improve their awareness, clarify their values and motivations, and improve their physical health. In this chapter, we will look at ways to use biophilia to support the well-being of individuals with dementia.

Nature-Based Interventions

Before I launch into ways to use biophilia-based tools to support and improve the well-being of our people with dementia, I'd like to share some thoughts about curiosity. Curiosity is a natural part of human and animal behavior. It is an intense desire for knowledge and exploration, and is often characterized by a sense of wonder and inquisitiveness about the world around us. Curiosity is important for personal growth and development, and can provide meaning and value throughout life, including for our people with dementia.

However, curiosity can decline due to a lack of stimulation and the progression of dementia, leading to apathy. This is particularly true for older adults who may experience mobility issues, cognitive decline, and physical frailty, which can limit opportunities for observation and exploration.

As the caregiver, you can help keep that sense of curiosity alive in your person. Engaging in activities that stimulate curiosity can increase the release of dopamine, the feel-good chemical, in the brain, which can increase the desire to learn and explore. Research has also shown that older adults with higher levels of curiosity tend to have better memory retention.

One way to stimulate curiosity and support personal growth is by providing opportunities for exploration and observation in nature. The natural world has a way of captivating our attention and fostering a sense of wonder and curiosity. I provide ideas on how to keep that spark going below. Some are free or affordable; some are expensive. Some work for mobile people; some cater to people with reduced mobility. As you peruse these ideas, I recommend that you focus on the activities that you yourself would find the most engaging. Your enthusiasm will translate to your person. I wish you happiness and joy as you explore some of these options.

Going outside: If your person with dementia is mobile, taking them out for some fresh air and nature can seem like a daunting task. There are so many things to remember and prepare—making sure they're dressed for the weather, grabbing the wheelchair or cane, packing any necessary medication or snacks, and let's not forget about the endless trips to the bathroom before leaving the house. And that's all before you even step foot outside! It can feel like more trouble than it's worth. But the benefits of spending time in nature are well worth the effort. So take a deep breath, gather your patience, and enjoy the great outdoors with your loved one. I offer ideas for activities toward the end of this chapter in a section called "Outdoor Activities."

If decreased mobility is an issue, or if you just don't have it in you to pack like you're visiting Mount Kilimanjaro, see if you can spend just a little time on a patio, deck, or park bench. Research shows that just sitting outside can have significant health benefits,[11] and I've seen first-hand the positive impact that nature can have on my own people with dementia. My mom, who was no longer speaking, always wore a big smile when I took her on neighborhood wheelchair rides. My late husband, Joe, loved going on nature walks and collecting interesting stones and tree bark to display on the windowsills. And my grandmother was always eager to "get out of this place," so we'd take a walk around the block and both come back feeling rejuvenated. Even my dad, who had limited mobility, found solace in sitting on the deck.

If your person can't get outside, you still have options. As a hospice volunteer, every one of my patients had a deep need to be outside, regardless of the weather or time of year. When they couldn't be outside, they wanted to see out the window.[12] If this sounds like your situation, I offer some tips below to bring nature into the house.

Indoor plants: Indoor plants can provide a variety of benefits for our people with dementia. Not only do plants look pretty and add some life to a room, but they also help purify the air by removing harmful chemicals like carbon monoxide and converting it to oxygen. Also, studies have shown that caring for plants can help reduce triggers and symptoms of dementia.[13] So why not get your green thumb on and start sprucing up your space with some plants? You can even involve your person in the fun by helping to choose and care for the plants. And if your loved one is a fan of the great outdoors but can't always go out, consider adding some window boxes, a windowsill herb garden, or even a terrarium with miniature plants to give them a little taste of nature from the comfort of their own home. Just try to avoid putting plants on the dining table—they might distract from the main attraction (the food).

Water elements: Water elements provide multisensory nature-based experiences, thereby promoting the well-being of you and your person.[14] These can be small or large, outdoor or indoor. Outdoor examples include rain chains, which replace gutters and can be enjoyed from windows or patios. These are available at home improvement stores and online retailers such as Amazon, Lowes, Home Depot, and Best Buy. Another possibility involves koi ponds, which provide an excellent opportunity to experience the presence of water, watch fish, and engage in feeding activities. Your local zoo or aquarium might have them, or you could look into having one installed in your yard.

Indoor possibilities include aquaria, which can be a fun activity for you and your person to do together. You can pick out fish and set up the tank, or if that seems like too much work, beta fish just need a jar and food. Another small indoor option is an indoor waterfall. These have been shown to promote relaxation and lower blood pressure.[15] Some of these are easy to install and offer soothing sounds, attractive lights, and the visual pleasure of falling water. Many fit on desks or shelves and can be easily purchased from home improvement stores or online retailers.

If your person struggles with incontinence, the sound of water might be unhelpful, and some people with dementia develop a deep fear of water, so this tool—like all others—isn't for everyone. However, if your person enjoys water, there are plenty of options to include a beneficial feature in their home or garden. A big indoor option is available through interactive projector technology (as discussed in chapter 8). The projector can add elements such as interactive koi ponds or interactive bird flocks to the walls and floors of your home, providing a nature-based experience without the need for cage cleaning.

Air: Air is an important natural element that can promote calm and enhance well-being. Fresh, natural ventilation is preferred over processed, stagnant air. The movement of air and the stimulation it provides, such as how it feels on the skin or the smell of the air after a rain, can be invigorating and healthy. To ensure good air quality in your home, make sure to open windows and provide access to outdoor areas such as porches, patios, and balconies. Ceiling fans can also help improve air circulation. It is important to pay attention to air filtration, humidity, and temperature control to prevent respiratory illness, especially during flu season.

Views of nature: Visual access to human activity, children playing, natural views of gardens, water elements, and wildlife like birds can be most satisfying. Even persons with late stages of dementia can be found gazing out the window for hours at a time.[16]

Improving views out of windows can be a simple yet effective way to provide stimulation and enjoyment for your person. Here are some ways to enhance the view:

- Clean the windows: Make sure windows are clean and unobstructed, so that your person has a clear view of the outside.
- Add window boxes or pots: Consider adding window boxes or pots filled with flowers or plants to the windowsill. This can provide a colorful and visually appealing view for your person. I add tiny seasonal decorations to one of my window boxes, and this provided a topic of conversation for me and my late husband.
- Install bird feeders: Bird feeders can attract a variety of birds and provide a visual and auditory experience for your loved one. Plus, watching the birds—and squirrels—at the feeder can be a great form of entertainment.
- Create a window garden: If your loved one enjoys gardening, consider creating a small window garden where they can tend to plants. This can provide a sense of purpose and accomplishment.
- Break out the binoculars: For a closer look at the great outdoors, try using binoculars. You can also consider purchasing a pair of binoculars specifically designed for people with vision impairments, which may have larger objective lenses and more comfortable eyepieces. Just be prepared for your loved one to spot things you never knew were there—like that one particularly interesting leaf on the tree across the street.

Overall, the simple act of looking out the window can provide a sense of connection to the natural world and bring joy to people with dementia.

Nature is filled with beautiful and distinct elements that draw our attention and serve as focal points. These focal points, such as mountains, unique trees, canyons, or ponds, help us orient ourselves and understand our surroundings. In our homes, it is important to have clear focal points as well, to help people with dementia understand the purpose and use of a room or space. For example, the front door of a house is a natural focal point, but if the entry to the home is hidden or difficult to find, it can cause confusion and make it difficult for a person with dementia to orient themselves. Similarly, each room should have a clear focal point, such as a bed in a bedroom or a fireplace in a living room. Identifying and highlighting these focal points can help support spatial understanding and reduce confusion for people with dementia. (See chapter 5, "Furnishings Matter," for more tips on creating effective focal points in your home.)

Animals: Pets, such as cats, dogs, fish, birds, rabbits, hamsters, and other small animals, can provide comfort and new meaning for people with dementia. The presence of animals and their stimulation of life is a powerful biophilic element that can provide love and nurturing for those who may be feeling lonely. Dogs and cats are particularly popular pets for dementia therapy. Research has shown that the presence of a dog can increase social interaction, reduce agitation, improve physical activity, increase pleasure, and improve eating in people with dementia. Dogs are highly social animals and are known for their ability to provide support and unconditional love, making them great companions and therapists for those with dementia. Studies have shown that the use of companion animals paired with people with dementia can increase socialization and decrease agitation behaviors, and can combat loneliness, stress, and depression. In the section below, I discuss the benefits of some animals to people with dementia and their caregivers.

Fish: Fish gazing, also known as aquatherapy, is a form of therapy that involves the use of fish tanks or aquariums as a form of visual stimulation for people with dementia. It is believed that the movement of the fish, as well as the bright colors and patterns of the fish and their surroundings, can help to improve mood, reduce agitation and anxiety, and potentially improve cognitive function in people with dementia.[17]

Where can you and your person with dementia get your fish-gazing fix, you ask? Well, here are a few options:

1. Therapy centers: Some therapy centers offer aquatherapy as part of their treatment programs for people with dementia. It's a great way

to get in some exercise and stimulation, all while enjoying the peaceful presence of some finned friends.

2. Community centers: Local community centers and senior centers may have fish tanks or aquariums that are available for people with dementia to visit and watch. It's a great way to get out of the house and enjoy some relaxing fish-watching time.

3. At home: If you have a green thumb and a love for fish, why not set up a small fish tank or aquarium at home for your person with dementia to enjoy? It's a great way for your person and you to relax and engage with a calming activity.

4. Zoos and aquariums: Your local zoo or aquarium might have programs for people with dementia, and you might be able to see monkeys and otters, too.

Birds: Birds have long been beloved pets in the home and backyard, and they are now being recognized for their therapeutic benefits in hospitals and senior living environments. People with dementia are often captivated by birds and can find watching them to be a peaceful, engaging, and enjoyable activity. The movement of birds as they build their nests, fly from branch to branch, and splash in a small bowl of water can help to ease anxiety and restlessness in people with dementia. Both outdoor habitats and indoor aviaries can be delightful places for people with dementia to watch and interact with birds.

The Audubon Society has developed an innovative program called Bird Tales that connects people with dementia to the world of birds. The program uses multisensory stimulation and the natural world of birds to improve outdoor habitats while also providing a meaningful and engaging experience for people with dementia. According to David Yarnold, president of the Audubon Society, "The Bird Tales program brings peace and joy to people living with dementia by connecting them with the healing power of birds." The program includes a training video and workbook that provide step-by-step instructions for creating bird-friendly habitats and engaging with birds in a therapeutic way. The Bird

Tales program is easily replicable at home and the workbook is available for purchase on the internet and on Amazon.

Dementia service dogs: The primary task of a dementia service dog is to keep your person with dementia safe. If your person is a wanderer, a service dog might be a great solution. Service dogs try to deter your person from leaving their home unaccompanied. If your person succeeds in slipping out the door, the dogs are equipped with GPS collars that allow the owner's family to locate them. Also, the dog is trained to bark constantly, grabbing the attention of any passersby. The dogs are also trained to assist with tasks such as waking your person up in the morning, reminding your person where their clothes are, and even bringing your person their medication in a bite-proof box. In addition to these practical services, dementia service dogs can also provide companionship and offer a listening ear. It's worth noting that while service dogs can be very helpful in addressing the needs of people with dementia, regular pets can also provide some of the same benefits, such as companionship, anxiety reduction, and opportunities for fresh air and exercise.

Service dogs are not a substitute for a caregiver. However, they can provide valuable support and improve the quality of life for both your person and you. There are several steps involved in getting a service dog for a person with dementia:

1. Determine if a service dog is the right solution for you.
2. Find a reputable service dog organization. Just because a group calls itself a "service dog organization" doesn't mean it's legitimate. Check for things like "accreditation," "standards," and "not being run out of a van in a Walmart parking lot."
3. Submit an application.
4. Go through the matching process. This is where the service dog organization will try to figure out what kind of dog would be the best fit for you. Just like when you're trying to pick out a new pair of

shoes—some dogs are comfortable, some are stylish, and some will just make your feet hurt.

5. Attend training. This is where you'll learn how to work with your new furry friend. Just remember: the dog is not a replacement for your caregiver, so don't try to make it do things like cook dinner or file your taxes.

6. Take the dog home and continue training.

Fire: Fire elements, such as fireplaces and candles, can provide warmth, heating, and a sense of comfort and calm. The hearth, or fireplace, is often seen as the heart of the home and can serve as a gathering place for family. Gazing into a flickering flame has been shown to shift brainwaves from a state of reactivity (beta state) to a state of relaxation (alpha brainwave state), which can help to relax the mind and make it more open and receptive. The warmth, glow, smells, and sounds associated with fire can also contribute to a feeling of comfort and calm.

Today, it is easy and inexpensive to add a fireplace or hearth to a home using electronic devices that mimic flames and even produce the sounds of burning wood. Fire elements can also be incorporated into outdoor grills or patios, and can provide a visually and sensory engaging backdrop for storytelling and reminiscing. Candles, which are also part of the fire element, can create a mood, celebrate a special occasion, or provide a warm ambiance. For safety, it is best to use realistic mock candles rather than open flames. Candles can be added to a holiday table or any festive living space to create a warm and inviting atmosphere.

Outdoor Activities

If your person is mobile, and if you have the energy and motivation, going outside provides abundant benefits. But what to do? I recommend finding nature-based destination that you yourself love and find engaging. Your person will be happier when you are happier. I offer some ideas below.

1. Gardening: Planting flowers, herbs, or vegetables can provide a sense of accomplishment and purpose, as well as an opportunity to get some gentle exercise and enjoy the outdoors. I discuss this in more detail below.

2. Nature walks: Taking a leisurely walk through a park or nature trail can be a relaxing and enjoyable way to get some fresh air and enjoy the beauty of nature. Sometimes even a walk through your backyard can help.

3. Bird watching: Watching birds and other wildlife can be a peaceful and engaging activity that stimulates the senses and promotes cognitive function.

4. Outdoor games: Simple games such as tossing a ball or frisbee, playing catch, or hitting a balloon back and forth can provide physical activity and a sense of playfulness. Consider taking a board or card game outside and play under a tree or on the patio or deck.

5. Picnics: Pack a lunch and head to a local park or beach for a relaxing outdoor meal.

6. Scenic drives: Going for a drive through a scenic area can provide a change of scenery and an opportunity to enjoy the beauty of the outdoors.

7. Sensory experiences: Engaging the senses through activities such as smelling flowers, listening to the sounds of nature, or feeling the warmth of the sun can be enjoyable and stimulating.

8. Your place of worship: When my mother with Parkinson's had meltdowns and I could not calm her, we would walk to her church and sit quietly in the back. Sometimes we would cry, but we both experienced a sense of calm.

9. Outdoor venues: Look for outdoor venues you and your person might enjoy together. Craft shows, art fairs, and fruit-picking excursions offer opportunities to get outside and see new things. My mom loved farm stands and insisted on buying a bushel of tomatoes to can for the winter, reminiscing about when she and my grandmother canned tomatoes for their family.

10. Try the beach: The benefits of aquatic exercise for those with dementia include improving functional capacity and significantly affect other aspects of quality of life such as sleep, appetite, behavioral

and psychological symptoms, depression, and falls. Additionally, swimming can improve a person's overall well-being and positively enhance sociality.[18]

11. Al fresco dining: Since the pandemic, many restaurants have expanded outdoor dining. Outdoor restaurants offer a comfortable choice for your person with dementia and are less confining than the indoor counterpart.

Gardens

Gardens can be a wonderful place for relaxation and interaction with nature. They offer a range of aesthetics, including the sights of colorful flowers and plants, the smells of fragrances, the sounds of birdsong, and the tactile experiences of touching garden elements. Gardens can be enjoyed by people of all cognitive abilities and are particularly appealing when they are visible from multiple locations, including windows.

Gardening has a number of benefits for our people with dementia, including supporting mobility and agility, stimulating cognitive function, and providing opportunities for reminiscing about past gardening experiences. When planning a garden, perhaps consider incorporating a variety of flowers, produce, green plants, and deciduous and evergreen shrubs of different sizes and colors. Edible plants, like cherry tomatoes, can be especially appealing. Be sure to include both active and passive activities, and provide areas with sun and shade. Water features, bird feeders, and fish ponds can add elements of nature and interest. Outdoor sculptures and comfortable, safe garden furniture can also provide pleasant visual attractions and places to rest and socialize.

Gardens can also be made dementia-friendly by ensuring they are easy to navigate, with smooth, low-glare paths that accommodate wheelchairs and have handrails for balance and security. Water gardens with colorful fish can provide sensory stimulation, and interactive gardens with raised beds, flower gardens, and other activities can encourage participation and socialization. Reminiscence gardens, which include familiar items from the past, can stimulate memories and conversations with family and friends. Wander gardens, which allow for free movement in a controlled, fenced area, have been shown to improve mood and quality of life for people with dementia.

Perhaps you can plant a simple garden yourself, or you can visit your local botanical garden. Your local community center might have ideas about local garden programs in support of our people with dementia. Overall, gardens can be a wonderful resource for relaxation, interaction with nature, and meaningful activities for people with dementia as well as their caregivers and families.

Prospect and Refuge

Prospect-refuge is a pattern derived from nature and used in the built environment. To goal is to provide (a) a clear view over a distance for surveillance and planning and (b) a place to withdraw from the main flow of activity. This pattern is important for human well-being and place attachment because it allows individuals to feel both protected and able to observe their surroundings. In architecture and landscaping, prospect can be provided through high vantage points, while refuge can be provided through edges of a scene or protected areas that allow for observation from a distance.

In long-term care facilities, designing spaces that incorporate both prospect and refuge can help create a sense of residential scale and non-institutionality, as well as provide a variety of spatial experiences for residents with different functional abilities and preferences. Examples of long-term care facilities that effectively balance prospect and refuge include the Leonard Florence Center for Living Green House in Boston and the Ørestad Retirement Home in Copenhagen. (See figure 9.1.)

To incorporate this concept into the home environment of a person with dementia, caregivers can:

1. Create clear views of the outside world from a protected vantage point, such as from a window or balcony.
2. Designate safe spaces in the home, such as a bedroom or quiet corner, that are free from potential hazards and provide a sense of privacy and security.

3. Use natural elements, such as plants or water features, to create a sense of refuge and a calming atmosphere.
4. Ensure proper lighting in key areas of the home to help the person feel safe and secure.
5. Consider the person's individual needs and preferences and adjust the home environment accordingly.

For example, my grandmother with dementia found comfort and security in hiding in my mother's bedroom closet during a noisy family holiday gathering. By understanding her individual needs and preferences, we could have created a home environment that provided a sense of prospect and refuge for her so that she didn't need to hide in the closet.

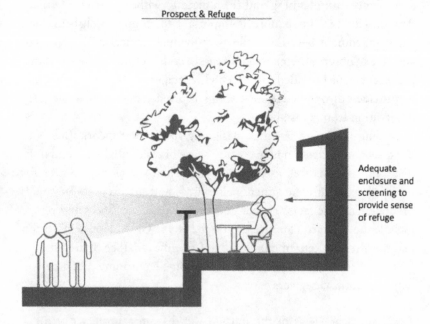

Prospect & Refuge

Adequate enclosure and screening to provide sense of refuge

FIGURE 9.1. SCHEMATIC DRAWING OF AN OUTDOOR PROSPECT REFUGE
Research shows that people with dementia feel safer and engaged when they can look out on the world without being easily visible themselves. We can lean on that information by creating prospect refuges for them, both indoors and outdoors. *Source:* Illustrated by Grace Boateng.

Figure 9.1 illustrates prospect and refuge. The concept of prospect and refuge refers to the feeling of protection and safety provided by certain environments. This is especially important for individuals with dementia, whose perception of threats and safety can be complex and difficult for caregivers to understand.

CONCLUSION

Nature has been my go-to intervention during my caregiving journeys. It has helped me just as much as it's helped my people with dementia. The positive distraction of nature has helped solve some of our most difficult challenges, meltdowns, and disruptive behaviors. Whether it's just going for a short walk outside or cuddling with the dog, nature has a way of resetting our stress levels. The possibilities for nature-based interventions are endless, and they can be incredibly effective.

Nature isn't a cure-all for the difficulties of dementia care, but when things feel chaotic and overwhelming, consider using nature as a distraction. She's a great friend to have in times of need. And the best part is, the joy of nature can be experienced by everyone—our people with dementia, their caregivers, and their families.

10

Sensory Engagement

The five senses are ministers of the soul.

—*Leonardo da Vinci*

In the late stages of Alzheimer's, my late father-in-law no longer knew his son's name or mine. He called us "those nice people," when he could find any words at all. He now lived in a memory care facility, incontinent and unable to do most activities of daily living. However, he was ambulatory and always enjoyed going to church with us. Dressed in his suit and tie with the help of caregivers, we picked him up and went to the church where things felt familiar and comfortable and he knew the liturgy.

Our church was rich in sensory stimulation: gold leaf icons, resonant chants, musical bells, flickering candles, and intensely fragrant incense. He had participated in this ritual since he was a small child. At church, my father-in-law didn't just sit there, as he did in most places. Here, he fully participated—kneeling, sitting, standing, even singing and chanting along with the congregation. His face became animated. Following the service, he sometimes even spoke with other parishioners, albeit briefly.

Once we left the church, he would retreat into his typical silence. The bounty of sensory input targeted deeply embedded memories, allowing his Sunday visits to bring him to life, if only for a brief time.

SENSES AND DEMENTIA

The human senses—sight, sound, smell, touch, and taste—play a crucial role in our ability to experience and interact with the world around us. These senses provide us with the means to communicate, work, feel pleasure and pain, and heal. They also serve as the gatekeepers to our consciousness, influencing our emotions and behavior.

Our senses are closely connected to our brain's pleasure and pain receptors and can influence our emotions,[1] but as we age or suffer from dementia-based diseases, our cognitive function can decline. Because our emotional responses often remain intact, sensory interventions provide effective ways to alleviate behavioral and psychological symptoms of dementia.[2] Sternberg[3] suggests that eliciting emotions, rather than focusing on cognitive function, may be a more compelling model for dementia interventions.

Our people with dementia may experience changes in their sense organs as the disease progresses, potentially leading to a reduction in sensory abilities. As caregivers, we can maximize access to their senses. After we've made sure that they can see, hear, taste, smell, and feel to the best of their ability, we can make sure that the world that they sense provides pleasure with the understanding that some noises, odors, or other sensory experiences may contribute to anxiety and undesirable behaviors. By being aware of and proactively addressing these issues, we can improve the emotional quality of life for our people and mitigate the adverse effects of the aging process on the senses.

In this chapter, I describe how dementia affects each of the senses, how we can lean on them to improve the lives of our people, and how we can protect them to reduce disruptive behaviors.

Vision

Sight is a crucial sense that allows us to perceive and understand the world around us. It allows us to classify and judge our surroundings. As caregivers, we can use our understanding of sight to help our people with dementia live more independent and meaningful lives.

Technically, the eye only sees pieces of an image. The brain puts these pieces together to form a whole picture. For example, when we look at an apple, the eye sees the individual lines and edges, but the brain recognizes the apple and associates it with memories of taste and pleasure. If the brain's abilities are in decline, the eye may still see the apple, but the pleasure of eating it may require the involvement of other senses, such as taste and smell. In fact, engaging multiple senses can often link memories and help with recognition.[4]

My mom had always been a big fan of apples, enjoying them as a snack or in pies. As her dementia progressed and I would offer her an apple, she seemed to not recognize it as a piece of edible fruit. I was surprised. She had turned so many of them into pies. She'd pulled them out of her purse on road trips. In my mind's eye, I could see her walking near the lake, crunching on an apple. I knew that her love for them was buried in her damaged brain. Finally, by engaging her sense of smell and linking it with the sight of the apple—I put a sliced apple and a whole apple on one plate—I was able to help her rediscover the pleasure of eating it. She'd eat it and tell me how good it was. But even after this rediscovery, she soon forgot the enjoyment of the apple, as the memory that associated it with pleasure was lost. The decline of cognitive function due to dementia can disrupt the connection between the senses and memories, but you might find ways to access it.

How the dementia eye sees: Dementia can affect vision in a number of ways. Some common changes that may occur include:

1. Decreased visual acuity: This refers to the ability to see small details clearly. People with dementia may have difficulty reading or seeing objects that are far away or up close.
2. Reduced visual field: The visual field is the area that can be seen while looking straight ahead. People with dementia may have a smaller visual field, which can make it difficult to see objects to the side or in the periphery. For people with dementia, they may see the world as if looking through binoculars.

3. Difficulty with color perception: Some people with dementia may have trouble distinguishing between different colors or may see colors differently than they used to.

4. Problems with depth perception: This refers to the ability to judge the distance and size of objects. As dementia advances, your person's brain may find that the information coming in through two eyes overwhelming, so it may shut down information coming from one eye. That makes it hard for your person to know if something is a pattern in the carpet or an object on the floor, a real apple or a picture of an apple, or what the chair seat's height is. They may have difficulty determining how far away objects are, which can make it hard to reach for or grab them.

5. Light sensitivity: Some people with dementia may become more sensitive to light or may have difficulty adapting to changes in lighting conditions.

6. Difficulty with eye movements: People with dementia may have trouble following moving objects with their eyes or may have difficulty making smooth eye movements. This can make it difficult to read or watch television.

Taken together, these changes in vision might drive behavior changes that don't make sense to us. Your person might act like they're picking at the air, but they're actually trying to turn off the ceiling light. Because they don't have depth perception, they don't know how far away the light really is. If your person starts picking at the air in front of them, they may be trying to pick something up off the floor. This type of behavior might look very strange to us, but your person may simply be responding to the world as they see it.

Please note that vision changes can vary widely among individuals with dementia, and some people may experience no changes at all. It is always a good idea to have regular eye exams to monitor for any changes in vision, and sometimes good glasses might alleviate strange behavior for a while.

Hearing

If you have hearing loss, you have a greater chance of developing dementia. In fact, researchers list hearing loss as one of the top risk factors for dementia. Even mild levels of hearing loss increase the long-term risks of cognitive decline and dementia.[5] The causal mechanism behind the relationship is not fully understood, but the leading hypotheses are:

- Hearing loss can make the brain work harder, forcing it to strain to hear and fill in the gaps. That comes at the expense of other thinking and memory systems.
- Hearing loss causes the aging brain to shrink more quickly.
- Hearing loss leads people to be less socially engaged, which is hugely important to remaining intellectually stimulated. If you can't hear very well, you may not go out as much, so the brain is less engaged and active.

Hearing loss has also been linked to social isolation, the risk of falls, depression, disability, lower quality of life, and increased healthcare costs.

However, there is good news! Hearing loss is a modifiable risk factor. That means, if you get hearing aids, you can prevent cognitive decline and dementia.[6] People with normal hearing and hearing aid users have similar risk of cognitive impairment, and quality audiology screening might prove an effective dementia prevention strategy.

As you are reading this book, if someone you care about is hard of hearing, urge them to get hearing aids—for their mental well-being and overall health. Get your person's hearing assessed, and get yours checked too. Medicaid covers them in some states, the prices for these devices are declining, and the quality is improving.

Music and People with Dementia

Universally, humans are passionate about music—and the theories behind this universality speak to ways to connect with our people with dementia. One idea suggests that music has a powerful effect on the brain, causing it to release feel-good chemicals such as endorphins;

this links music to strong emotional impacts that can trigger memories and feelings. A second theory suggests that music evolved as a way for humans to bond and communicate with one another. Regardless of the cause, people express deep emotions and share experiences though music, and it has been a central part of human culture and society for thousands of years.

Through music, you might be able to reach your person with dementia when words fail. Long-term memory for music is stored in a different part of the brain than other types of memories such as ordinary memories or language. The supplementary motor cortex, which is responsible for complex motor movements, serves as the storage location for long-term music memory, and this area of the brain is less affected by the typical metabolic disorders and nerve cell loss that occur in dementia. As a result, long-term music memory is often preserved in people with dementia, even as their other memories and cognitive functions decline.[7] The ability to access music—and its associated memories and emotions—may endure in people with dementia, even as their brains fail.

In this section, I'm going to discuss music therapy and music-based interventions, what we know about these approaches from research, and how you can apply them to your life and the life of your person.

Music therapy: The American Music Therapy Association defines music therapy as "the clinical and evidence-based use of music interventions to accomplish individualized goals within a therapeutic relationship by a certified individual who has completed an approved music therapy program." Music therapy helps people with dementia engage more actively with their environment and to better express their emotions. Although dementia is characterized as a disturbance of higher cortical functions (such as memory, thinking, and judgment), people with dementia can often still remember the lyrics of songs they learned as children. In fact, long-term music memory is better preserved than short-term memory, autobiographical long-term memory, or language.[8]

A person certified in music therapy, a music therapist, will develop music therapy treatment plans specific to the needs and strengths of the client, who may be seen individually or in groups. Music therapy treatment plans are individualized for each client. This means that the goals, objectives, and potential strategies of the music therapy services are appropriate for the individual client and setting. The music therapy interventions may include music improvisation, receptive music listening, song writing, lyric discussion, music and imagery, singing, music performance, learning through music, music combined with other arts, music-assisted relaxation, music-based patient education, electronic music technology, adapted music intervention, and movement to music.

Music therapy can be beneficial for people with dementia in several ways. It can improve their overall cognition, memory, and language skills, and reduce behavioral and psychological symptoms of dementia such as anxiety, depression, and agitation. Music therapy can also improve mood and social interactions, and provide a sense of accomplishment and enjoyment. It may also have physiological benefits, such as reducing blood pressure and heart rate. Music therapy can be a useful complement to other forms of treatment and can be tailored to individual needs and preferences. In short, the use of music therapy in people with dementia can help improve the perceived quality of life and well-being and may delay the progress of the disorder.[9]

To find a certified music therapist, I recommend that you start with the internet. The American Music Therapy Association is a great place to start.

Music-based interventions: While music therapy involves the use of music by a trained and certified therapist to address the needs of individuals, music-based interventions are more casual and not usually led by a trained and certified therapist. Music-based interventions are considered more a leisure activity than a therapeutic intervention.

Music-based interventions may be used for a variety of purposes, such as entertainment or socialization, and are not necessarily designed to be therapeutic or to achieve specific goals.

As the caregiver, you know what music is most meaningful to your person. Individualized music is important in both music therapy and music-based interventions.

There are several ways to implement music-based interventions at home for your person with dementia. Here are a few examples:

1. Play the person's favorite music: Creating a playlist of the person's favorite music can help to stimulate their memories and emotions.
2. Sing along: Singing along to familiar songs can be a fun and engaging activity for people with dementia. It can also help to improve mood and reduce stress.
3. Play musical instruments: Encourage the person to play a musical instrument, or play together as a group. This can be a fun and therapeutic activity for people with dementia.
4. Use music as a background activity: Playing music in the background during daily activities can help to create a pleasant and calming atmosphere.

You can also tie these interventions to other activities to make the impact stronger. Here are some examples:

1. Use music-based interventions as part of a sensory stimulation program. For example, you can play music that is related to a specific theme or activity, such as music from a particular era or music that evokes a particular place or activity, while eating meals or dressing in clothes from that era.
2. Music-based interventions can be used to promote movement and physical activity in people with dementia. For example, you can play music with a strong beat or rhythm and encourage your loved one to dance or move to the music. Wearing clothes that match the dance or exercise and joining your person might further the impact.

3. Music-based interventions can also be used to stimulate cognitive function. For example, you can play music that requires the listener to think critically, such as music with complex rhythms, lyrics, or melodies. These will work best if the music comes from the time period when your person was a teen or young adult.
4. Music-based interactions can be used to encourage social interaction. For example, you can play music that encourages singing or playing instruments together, or you can use music as a way to encourage conversation and reminiscing about past experiences.

Benefits of individualized music-based interventions have positive physiological, psychological, and emotional impacts. Music is good medicine with no side effects.

Examples from my own life: Theoretical lists are one thing, but I found in my own journeys with my people with dementia that I was often able to use music-based interventions effectively. (I didn't know about music therapy and its associated benefits at the time, although I really wish I had.) I provide some mini vignettes below. Maybe one will inspire you.

- Following an outburst where she threw books, I was able to bring my mom back to herself by singing familiar Christmas carols. They soothed her spirits, distracted her, and soon she joined me. It was August.
- When my late husband was in hospice, he would tap his toe to a beat and sing along under his breath while listening to a playlist he and his granddaughter had built.
- As I described in the opening story, my father-in-law, who was in late-stage dementia and unable to speak, sang the entire church liturgy when we brought him to church.
- When my mom was in hospice and had been unable to speak for months, I put on music from World War II. When one song started, she opened her eyes and said, "That's Sarah Vaughan." She sang along.

- A priest friend regularly visited his long-time parishioner Elenore in a memory care unit. She was often anxious and rebellious and refused to participate whenever he offered her Communion. During the Easter season, he came to her bedside singing the Easter chant. The song reached her where his words could not. Elenore joined the chant and participated in the sacrament. After seeing the effect music had on his visit, my friend entered the rooms of all of his dementia congregants with a song or chant.
- My mom, with late-stage Parkinson's, was unable to participate in any daily activities. When I played "The Bugle Boy of Company B," she was able to dress herself.
- My late husband had been an accomplished musician. In mid-stage dementia, he surprised our Christmas party guests. Although he couldn't remember his friends' names, he picked up a violin and played Christmas music perfectly. People with music training can continue to play music even as cognition declines.
- With a tube in her throat and no longer speaking, hospice patient Helen smiled while listening to her favorite waltzes hours before her last breath.

Laughter

Laughter has a number of physiological benefits that can improve overall health and well-being. Some of these benefits include relaxation, increased blood flow, reduced blood pressure, improved immune system function, pain relief, improved mental function, and improved social connections.

Laughter has the ability to relax the whole body and reduce feelings of stress and anxiety. It can also increase blood flow, which can be beneficial for cardiovascular health. In addition, laughter has been shown to reduce blood pressure, making it useful for individuals with hypertension.

The immune system can also be boosted by laughter, as it has been shown to increase the production of antibodies and stimulate the production of immune cells. Laughter has also been found to be an effective natural painkiller, as it increases the production of endorphins that help to reduce pain perception.

Importantly for our people with dementia, laughter has been shown to improve brain function, including increasing the production of brain-derived neurotrophic factor (BDNF), a protein that supports the survival of nerve cells. Evidence from care facilities supports this. Researchers recently found a link between a greater variety of occasions for laughter and a lower risk of dementia in Japanese older adults. The study also found that laughing during conversations with friends, communicating with children or grandchildren, and listening to the radio were primarily associated with a decreased risk of dementia. Their findings suggest that laughter may actually be protective against dementia and that engaging in a variety of laughter-inducing activities may be beneficial.[10]

So how do you get your person to laugh? My first suggestion is wait until you're in the mood to laugh yourself. If you don't see that on the near horizon, consider recruiting one of your belly-laughing friends. Below is a list of other ideas:

1. Share funny stories or jokes. Reminiscing about past experiences or telling jokes can be a good way to bring a smile to someone's face.
2. Engage in activities with a humorous element. Doing activities that are inherently funny, such as playing a silly game or acting out a skit, can be a good way to bring joy to someone with dementia.
3. Use humor to defuse difficult situations. Sometimes, using humor can help to alleviate tension or discomfort in difficult situations. For example, if someone with dementia is feeling anxious or agitated, making a silly face or telling a joke may help to defuse the situation and bring a smile to their face.
4. Use props or costumes. Using props or costumes can add a playful element to an activity and may help to bring a sense of levity to a situation.
5. Encourage laughter and smiling. Sometimes, simply encouraging a person with dementia to laugh or smile can help to bring joy to their

day. For example, you could play a game where you try to make each other laugh, or encourage the person with dementia to smile by smiling yourself.

It's important to keep in mind that what brings laughter and joy to one person with dementia may not work for another. But you know your person best. Things that made them laugh when they were young might still work. Fart jokes, anyone?

Touch

Touch is a sense that allows us to experience the world in a profound and intimate way. It allows us to feel the softness of a flower petal, the smoothness of a piece of glass, or the warmth of a hug. Through touch, we can communicate our emotions, offer comfort, and establish connections with others. The sense of touch is essential to our well-being and plays a vital role in how we perceive and interact with the world around us. Whether it is the gentle caress of a lover or the comforting pat on the back from a friend, touch has the power to bring us closer together and enrich our lives in countless ways.

Touch therapy, also known as massage therapy, is a form of alternative medicine that involves the use of touch to manipulate the soft tissues of the body. It is based on the idea that touch can have therapeutic benefits and can be used to promote relaxation, reduce stress, and improve circulation. Massage therapists use a variety of techniques, including kneading, rubbing, and pressing, to manipulate the muscles, tendons, and other soft tissues of the body. Massage therapy is often used to treat muscle tension, pain, and other physical problems, and is also believed to have emotional and psychological benefits.

Touch can have many therapeutic benefits for people with dementia, including reducing anxiety, promoting relaxation, and improving mood. In addition to these emotional benefits, touch can also have physical benefits such as lowering cortisol levels, which is a stress hormone, and improving sleep quality and the immune system. Massage therapy can be particularly effective for people with dementia, as it involves the gentle manipulation of the muscles and soft tissues of the body. Research has shown that massage therapy can reduce the frequency and intensity of agitated behavior in people with dementia.

There are many ways that caregivers can use touch to provide comfort and support to our people with dementia. Holding hands, giving a gentle shoulder touch, and hugging or kissing on the forehead can all communicate love and care. Manicures, pedicures, and other forms of personal care that involve gentle touch can also be beneficial. It is important to keep in mind that everyone is different and may have different preferences when it comes to touch, but you know your person best. What they liked before their disease will still be appreciated. Some people with dementia may be uncomfortable with certain types of touch, so it is important to be respectful of their boundaries and to communicate with them about what they are comfortable with.

In addition to the direct benefits of touch, therapeutic touch can also help strengthen relationships and facilitate well-being for both caregivers and people with dementia. It can help to build trust, convey acceptance, and provide reassurance. In one study, the professional caregivers in a nursing facility reported that they themselves felt better after giving massages to the people in their care.[11] Overall, touch can be a powerful tool for promoting physical and emotional well-being in people with dementia.

Taste and Smell

Taste and smell are two of the most fundamental and important senses that we possess. They play a vital role in our enjoyment of food and drink and help us to recognize and identify different flavors and aromas. The sense of taste is mediated by taste buds on the tongue and allows us to recognize the basic tastes of sweet, sour, salty, bitter, and umami. The sense of smell is mediated by receptors in the nose and allows us to recognize and distinguish a wide range of odors. Together, taste and smell allow us to fully experience the pleasures of food and drink and play a crucial role in our overall health and well-being.

Changes in a person's sense of taste and smell can be caused by a variety of factors, including aging, certain medications, and underlying health conditions. These changes can make food seem less appealing or may cause a person to lose interest in eating altogether.

People with dementia may experience changes in their eating habits, including a decrease in appetite, difficulty swallowing, changes in taste and smell, and changes in the ability to recognize and enjoy food. These changes can lead to malnutrition, weight loss, and difficulty with meal preparation. Caregivers should be aware of these changes and may need to provide easy-to-eat foods or assist with meals. It is important to encourage the person with dementia to eat a well-balanced diet and to seek the guidance of a healthcare professional if there are concerns about nutrition.

The act of eating involves more than just the taste of food. It also includes the preparation, cooking, presentation, and sharing of meals with others. Food can have a powerful effect on our mood, thoughts, motivations, and performance, and certain meals can either lift our spirits or bring us down. Foods that are high in sugar and carbohydrates can relax us by releasing insulin and regulating serotonin, while spices can stimulate us. Chocolate and cheese contain PEA, a chemical that our bodies produce when we are in love.

Our sense of smell plays a vital role in the pleasure we derive from food. When we smell something delicious, like freshly brewed coffee, our olfactory organ (located in the nose) detects the odor molecules and initiates a neural response. This response is then combined with our sense of taste, allowing us to experience the full flavor of the food. In fact, our sense of smell is even more powerful than our sense of taste—it takes more than 25,000 molecules of cherry pie to taste it but only a few to smell it.[12]

Dementia can impair a person's ability to smell and taste, which can lead to a loss of interest in eating and drinking. This can lead to weight loss and malnutrition, as well as the consumption of rotting leftovers or a diet that is too heavy in sweets (the only things that can be tasted). It is important to find creative ways to ensure that a person with dementia is still able to eat a healthy diet.

There are some things you can do to keep your person safe while meeting their dietary needs:

1. Use strong flavors and spices to add interest to meals. Since a person with dementia may have a reduced sense of taste, using bold flavors can help make meals more appealing.
2. Use visual cues to make meals more appealing. Plating food in an attractive way, using colorful fruits and vegetables, and adding garnishes can all help to make food more appealing to someone with dementia.
3. Encourage the person to eat with others. Sharing meals with others can be a social and enjoyable experience, which may help to increase appetite.
4. Offer a variety of foods and textures. Different people have different preferences, so it's important to offer a range of foods to see what the person with dementia enjoys.
5. Be patient and understanding. It can be frustrating if a person with dementia refuses to eat or seems disinterested in food. It's important to be patient and try to find ways to make meals enjoyable for them.
6. Consider using assistive devices. There are a variety of assistive devices that can make it easier for a person with dementia to eat, such as adapted utensils or special cups with lids.
7. Consult with a healthcare professional. If you are concerned about the person's nutrition or weight loss, it's important to consult with a healthcare professional for guidance on how to manage these issues.
8. You know your person. If they're refusing to eat an old standby, ensure that it's prepared the usual way.
9. Check your refrigerator. One day your person will know not to eat that old yogurt, and the next day they'll have no idea.

Disruptive behaviors: Your person's favorite foods may radically change as the disease progresses. Once a gourmet sushi expert, Joe refused any fish; his new favorites became hot dogs and mac and cheese.

There are several reasons why people with dementia may experience changes in their food preferences. Dementia can affect the brain's ability to perceive and process flavors, which can make food seem less appealing. Changes in taste and smell can also contribute to this. In addition, dementia can affect a person's ability to recognize and enjoy food, which can further decrease their appetite. Some people with dementia may become more selective in their food choices and may refuse to eat certain foods or only want to eat very specific foods. This may be due to changes in their ability to process information and make decisions, as well as changes in their preferences and habits. All of these things can lead to unhappy mealtimes.

Joe loved oatmeal for breakfast. A caregiver prepared oatmeal for him, but he wouldn't eat it. As I was leaving for work and saw his un-eaten breakfast, I asked if he was hungry. He indicated he was. I pushed the bowl toward him, and he pushed it away. I looked at it and noticed it was missing the cinnamon sugar. When I added it, he ate it. He didn't have the words to tell the caregiver, and only I—his person—knew this detail. These small details can contribute to nutritional health as well as the pleasure of taste.

Missing these personal preferences can also lead to disruptive behaviors. Your person may throw their cup or dish. Your person will not know how to communicate these details, yet these very details can make for nutritional success and a happier mealtime experience. If one is not eating well, one can be tense, agitated, and disruptive.

Here are some strategies that may help reduce disruptive behavior during mealtimes for someone with dementia:

- Maintain a regular routine. Having regular mealtimes and snacks can help the person with dementia feel more comfortable and reduce anxiety.
- Create a calm atmosphere. A quiet, relaxed environment can help reduce disruptive behavior during meals.
- Make food visually appealing. Using color-contrasted dinnerware and serving food in an attractive way can make it more appealing to the person with dementia.

- Use utensils with large, easy-to-hold handles. This can make it easier for the person with dementia to eat and reduce frustration.
- Offer finger foods. Allowing the person with dementia to feed themselves can give them a sense of control and reduce disruptive behavior.
- Encourage socialization. Eating with others, such as family members or caregivers, can provide a sense of companionship and encourage the person with dementia to eat.
- Provide assistance as needed. If the person with dementia is having difficulty feeding themselves, it may be helpful to provide assistance, such as cutting up food or spoon feeding.
- Consider using meal delivery programs. These can provide a variety of food options and make mealtimes easier for caregivers.
- Seek the guidance of a healthcare professional. If disruptive behavior during mealtimes is a persistent issue, it may be helpful to seek the advice of a healthcare professional, such as a doctor or a registered dietitian.

Aromatherapy: Aromatherapy is the use of essential oils, which are concentrated plant extracts, for therapeutic purposes. Some people believe that certain essential oils can have a positive effect on a person's mood and well-being and may be used as a complementary treatment for various health conditions, including dementia.

There is some limited evidence to suggest that certain essential oils may have a positive effect on behavior and cognitive function in people with dementia. For example, studies have shown that the use of lavender essential oil may help reduce agitation and improve sleep in people with dementia. Other essential oils that have been studied for their potential benefits in dementia include lemon, peppermint, and rosemary.

It is important to note that the use of essential oils in people with dementia should be approached with caution, as some oils can be toxic if ingested or applied to the skin undiluted. It is also important to consult a healthcare professional before using essential oils, as they may interact with medications or have other potential risks.

Sensory Stimulation

Sensory stimulation is the activation or stimulation of one or more senses. It can improve mood, encourage engagement, and provide a sense of pleasure and meaning in everyday life. For people with dementia, sensory stimulation can also help to provide a way to express themselves beyond words and improve self-esteem and well-being. Sensory stimulation therapies may include music, vibrations, lighting, aroma, graphic projections, textures, and pillows.

However, it is important to be aware that high levels of sensory stimulation can trigger disruptive behaviors, agitation, and aggression, while low levels can lead to wandering and rummaging. Environmental factors such as noise, clutter, and busyness can contribute to confusion and disruptive behavior. Strategies to reduce sensory overload may include decreasing noise levels, shielding windows from external noise, scheduling times for household cleaning, and using thermal and acoustic window coverings.

The sensory stimulation theory, developed by Laird in 1985, posits that effective learning occurs through the stimulation of the senses, with vision being the most important at 75 percent, followed by hearing at 13 percent, and smell, taste, and touch at 12 percent.[13] Research has also shown that sensory stimulation can enhance cognitive function. The Snoezelen concept, developed in the Netherlands in the 1970s, involves creating multisensory environments or spaces to provide a calming respite for people with dementia. These rooms may include light, color, sound, scent, and a combination of materials.[14]

The Snoezelen concept involves creating a multisensory environment or space to provide a calming respite for people with dementia. Here are some tips for bringing the Snoezelen concept into your home:

- Choose a quiet, private space: Select a room or area of your home that is quiet and free from distractions.
- Incorporate sensory elements: Use sensory elements such as light, color, sound, scent, and a combination of materials to create a sooth-

ing atmosphere. This may include items such as calming music, scented candles, soft blankets, and colorful pillows.

- Keep the space uncluttered: Avoid clutter or unnecessary objects that may be confusing or distracting.
- Encourage relaxation: Encourage the person with dementia to relax and engage with the sensory elements at their own pace.
- Seek guidance: If you are interested in implementing the Snoezelen concept at home, it may be helpful to seek guidance from a healthcare professional, such as a doctor or occupational therapist. They can provide additional recommendations and help you tailor the sensory environment to the needs of the person with dementia.

Effective sensory stimulation should be tailored to the individual, with an emphasis on the person rather than the therapy. Human interaction and activities that involve the person's interests can be particularly effective. For example, a foot massage before bedtime may not only help the person with dementia sleep better, but the closeness and touch of the caregiver can also provide a sense of comfort and understanding.

CONCLUSION

Connecting with your person with dementia through the five senses can be a meaningful and rewarding experience. Using the senses of sight, sound, touch, taste, and smell can help to create a sense of connection and understanding, and can also provide a sense of pleasure and comfort. Sharing a favorite meal or dessert, listening to music together, or holding hands can all be simple yet powerful ways to connect with someone with dementia. Incorporating sensory elements into activities and spending time together can help to strengthen the bond between you and your person, and can provide a sense of joy and meaning in the face of the challenges of the disease.

Conclusion

My ideas have undergone a process of emergence by emergency.
When they are needed badly enough, they are accepted.

—*R. Buckminster Fuller*

My mother lived for more than six years with dementia from Parkin-son's—she lived in her home for more than half that time. She was mobile. She was creative. She painted and created art. She would feed the birds and scold the squirrels. She walked to church, hung out with her family, and played with grandkids and great grandkids. She cooked her special-ties and spent hours giggling about funny stories with us. She would get on airplanes to visit her far-flung family. Hallucinations came and went, some with terror and others comical. Although she was slipping into the unknown darkness, she was mostly satisfied, happy, and dearly loved.

As her journey continued, Maxcine became easily agitated, especially when it came to her house. She couldn't enter her own home without resorting to disruptive behavior. She'd refuse to enter and insist it wasn't hers. She wanted a house and a home that no longer existed—the one she shared with her mother and siblings as a child.

Sometimes we blundered into helpful positive distractions that would nudge her back to herself. Taking a different path, changing the conversation, and singing to her sometimes soothed her stress and distracted her. Only then were we able to walk into her home easily.

The day came when she slipped too far into that unknown. She chased out the professional caregivers. She pushed away the people who knew her and adored her. She confused chaos with reality. Mom didn't transition gracefully to the memory care facility.

Even in the hands of professional caregivers, mom couldn't let go of her concept of home. After multiple escape attempts and initiating a coup to get the other residents to escape with her, she was kicked out of assisted living.

Throughout this process, we all struggled and suffered. We tried to reason with her. We tried to use the same logic we'd used on all of our children. We lost out tempers and, as her family, we became harsh. Nothing seemed to work. Of course it didn't. We didn't speak the language of dementia, we didn't meet other families going through similar events, we didn't get help. We didn't know that arguing would never change the outcome.

Maxcine was craving love and the familiar. She wanted her family to laugh with her, to help her remember those funny stories, to go to church with her, but, above all, to be kind. We didn't know how to do that for the woman who suddenly thought that hard-boiled eggs belonged in her tea. Maxcine longed for the human touch, the hug, the reassurance that everything would be okay. Sometimes we gave her lectures instead, berating her for her thoughtlessness.

Here's the thing I learned as a hospice volunteer. We think the end of our journey is tragic. It becomes the family focus, the goal we all gather around. But our people have had long and rich and interesting lives. The dementia part is only a short chapter. Maxcine herself had a long and happy life, even with dementia.

In her very last days, I sat at her bedside, playing her beloved big band music, hoping she could hear it. I held her hand, not knowing if she could feel my touch. I knew I'd never have another conversation with her. It was tempting, as I sat there, to dwell on the horrible way dementia had robbed her.

But she had lived a larger-than-life life, and remembering those parts suddenly seemed more important. She and my dad had actually climbed to the top of the presidents' heads at Mount Rushmore. She'd earned a scholarship to art school. She'd bought and run a large hotel, building the bar and restaurant into the best in a sixty-mile radius. As a young woman, she'd answered the door once wearing strategically placed coconuts and a banana. She'd been expecting her friends, but it was the local priest.

I had learned to speak dementia better by the time I accompanied Joe on his journey. He lived with mid-stage Alzheimer's for four years before heart disease took him. He passed in the family room of his dream house surrounded by the people who loved him best and his little dog. As an architect and lover of music, photography, art, and design, these pleasures stayed with him until his very last days.

For Joe, reminiscence intervention was the most successful, and I had learned how to implement well. If I put boxes of photos in front of him, he would sift through the images for hours. He couldn't tell me who was in most of the photos, but I had learned that it didn't matter.

Being highly social, he really enjoyed parties. Losing the ability to communicate frustrated him and could trigger him to throw objects. I had learned that positive distractions could prevent his outbursts. I could hand him his camera, put a drink in his hand, or give him a hug, thereby offsetting his frustration. I had also learned to stay with him since he would wander and get lost.

Nature walks by the river were my favorite pastime with him. Together with our little dog, we would wander. Joe would take pictures, and we would find a bench to sit on. Sometimes we'd reminisce, sometimes we'd sit quietly hand in hand, or sometimes we'd throw a stick for our puppy.

Joe also responded to music-based interventions. His granddaughter had made him a playlist of his favorite tunes. They had formed a close bond, choosing the music. When he became agitated, I would give him the headset, and he would lay back, smile, and listen. On Thursday nights, we would go to his favorite Greek restaurant, where they had live music. He would clap his hands, tap his toe, and sometimes even dance. He was no longer able to order from the menu and often played with his food, but music always brought him great pleasure.

Three days before he passed, he danced to the live music there.

THE END

Throughout this book, I have shared the problematic and challenging symptoms of my beloved people with dementia. I bumbled and struggled with the first journeys and became better at it for the last. I wrote this book thinking about my young self, telling her the things that would have made her life easier. I hope that some of these interventions work for you or that these inspire you to invent some of your own.

Like myself, the family caregiver often arrives to this role without training, resources, and experience. We are the sons, daughters, spouses, or friends. We are devastated by their diagnosis.

One of the hardest lessons I learned is that our people with dementia are not like toddlers. Sometimes we will think that they are. But toddlers learn and can be reasoned with. Brain damage prevents that in our people with dementia. Living in the moment, they forget your conversation or reprimands as soon as you walk away. They won't learn from their disruptive behaviors—but we can. I know I did.

Here is the last piece of advice I'd give my young self. Don't argue. Don't humor. Capitulate to the best of your ability. It isn't weakness; it's strength. When your person feels heard and valued, even when what they are saying seems crazy, they will feel less stress and less fear. And so will you. When that wolf comes to your door, you can still face it together.

Notes

INTRODUCTION

1. Alzheimer's Association, Facts and Figures Report (2022), www.alz.org.

2. Anke Jakob and Lesley Collier, "Sensory Enrichment for People Living with Dementia: Increasing the Benefits of Multisensory Environments in Dementia Care Through Design," *Design for Health* 1, no. 1 (2017): 115–33.

3. J. Tilly, "Responding to the Wandering and Exit-Seeking Behaviors of People with Dementia," *Journal of the American Geriatrics Society* 59 (2015): 473–81.

4. Barry Resiberg, Sunnie Kenowsky, Emile H. Franssen, Stefanie R. Auer, and Liduïn E. M. Souren, "Towards a Science of Alzheimer's Disease Management: A Model Based upon Current Knowledge of Retrogenesis," *International Psychogeriatrics* 11, no. 1 (1999): 7–23.

5. Bryce Carsone Smith and Mariana D'Amico, "Sensory-Based Interventions for Adults with Dementia and Alzheimer's Disease: A Scoping Review," *Occupational Therapy in Health Care* 34, no. 3 (2020): 171–201.

6. Aishah Diyana Baharudin, Normah Che Din, Ponnusamy Subramaniam, and Rosdinom Razali, "The Associations Between Behavioral-Psychological Symptoms of Dementia (BPSD) and Coping Strategy, Burden of Care and

Personality Style among Low-Income Caregivers of Patients with Dementia," *BMC Public Health* 19, no. 4 (2019): 1–12.

7. M. Uri Wolf, Yael Goldberg, and Morris Freedman, "Aggression and Agitation in Dementia," *Continuum: Lifelong Learning in Neurology* 24, no. 3 (2018): 783–803.

8. Po-Heng Tsai, "Clinical Management of Episodic Memory Changes in Dementia," *Current Treatment Options in Neurology* 20, no. 3 (2018): 1–11.

9. Marie A. Mills and Peter G. Coleman, "Nostalgic Memories in Dementia—A Case Study," *The International Journal of Aging and Human Development* 38, no. 3 (1994): 203–19.

10. Silvia M. Gramegna, "Reminiscence and Nostalgia: The Role of Design in the Development of Feasible Solutions for Dementia Care," in *Meanings of Design in the Next Era: 4D Osaka Conference Proceedings* (2019): 48–54.

CHAPTER 1

1. EunKyo Kang, Bhumsuk Keam, Na-Ri Lee, Jung Hun Kang, Yu Jung Kim, Hyun-Jeong Shim, Kyung Hae Jung, et al., "Impact of Family Caregivers' Awareness of the Prognosis on Their Quality of Life/Depression and Those of Patients with Advanced Cancer: A Prospective Cohort Study," *Supportive Care in Cancer* 29, no. 1 (2021): 397–407.

2. Julita Sansoni, Kathryn H. Anderson, Leydis M. Varona, and Graciela Varela, "Caregivers of Alzheimer's Patients and Factors Influencing Institutionalization of Loved Ones: Some Considerations on Existing Literature," *Ann Ig* 25, no. 3 (2013): 235–46.

3. Anu Berg, Heikki Palomäki, Jouko Lönnqvist, Matti Lehtihalmes, and Markku Kaste, "Depression among Caregivers of Stroke Survivors," *Stroke* 36, no. 3 (2005): 639–43.

4. Richard Schulz and Scott R. Beach, "Caregiving as a Risk Factor for Mortality: The Caregiver Health Effects Study," *JAMA* 282, no. 23 (1999): 2215–19.

5. Abby C. King, Roberta K. Oka, and Deborah R. Young, "Ambulatory Blood Pressure and Heart Rate Responses to the Stress of Work and Caregiving in Older Women," *Journal of Gerontology* 49, no. 6 (1994): M239–45.

6. Richard Holicky, "Caring for the Caregivers: The Hidden Victims of Illness and Disability," *Rehabilitation Nursing* 21, no. 5 (1996): 247–52.

7. World Health Organization Ageing and Life Course Unit, and Université de Genève Centre Interfacultaire de Gérontologie, *A Global Response to Elder Abuse and Neglect: Building Primary Health Care Capacity to Deal with the Problem World-Wide: Main Report* (Geneva: World Health Organization, 2008).

8. Lopez Hartmann, Maja, Johanna De Almeida Mello, Sibyl Anthierens, Anja Declercq, Thérèse Van Durme, Sophie Cès, Véronique Verhoeven, Johan Wens, Jean Macq, and Roy Remmen, "Caring for a Frail Older Person: The Association Between Informal Caregiver Burden and Being Unsatisfied with Support from Family and Friends," *Age and Ageing* 48, no. 5 (2019): 658–64.

9. Amy Horowitz, "Family Caregiving to the Frail Elderly," *Annual Review of Gerontology and Geriatrics* 5, no. 1 (1985): 194–246.

10. Norm O'Rourke, Philippe Cappeliez, and Sophie Guindon, "Depressive Symptoms and Physical Health of Caregivers of Persons with Cognitive Impairment: Analysis of Reciprocal Effects over Time," *Journal of Aging and Health* 15, no. 4 (2003): 688–712.

11. Josefine Persson, Lukas Holmegaard, Ingvar Karlberg, Petra Redfors, Katarina Jood, Christina Jern, Christian Blomstrand, and Gunilla Forsberg-Wärleby, "Spouses of Stroke Survivors Report Reduced Health-Related Quality of Life Even in Long-Term Follow-Up: Results from Sahlgrenska Academy Study on Ischemic Stroke," *Stroke* 46, no. 9 (2015): 2584–90.

12. Sonia J. Lupien, Robert-Paul Juster, Catherine Raymond, and Marie-France Marin, "The Effects of Chronic Stress on the Human Brain: From Neurotoxicity, to Vulnerability, to Opportunity," *Frontiers in Neuroendocrinology* 49 (2018): 91–105.

13. Maria Fernanda B. Sousa, Raquel L. Santos, Oriol Turró-Garriga, Rachel Dias, Marcia C. N. Dourado, and Josep L. Conde-Sala, "Factors Associated with Caregiver Burden: Comparative Study Between Brazilian and Spanish Caregivers of Patients with Alzheimer's Disease (AD)," *International Psychogeriatrics* 28, no. 8 (2016): 1363–74.

14. Barbara Huelat and Sharon T. Pochron, "Stress in the Volunteer Caregiver: Human-Centric Technology Can Support Both Caregivers and People with Dementia," *Medicina* 56, no. 6 (2020): 257.

15. Hideyuki Terayama, Hirofumi Sakurai, Nayuta Namioka, Rieko Jaime, Koko Otakeguchi, Raita Fukasawa, Tomohiko Sato, et al., "Caregivers' Education Decreases Depression Symptoms and Burden in Caregivers of Patients with Dementia," *Psychogeriatrics* 18, no. 5 (2018): 327–33.

16. Michelle Devor and Marian Renvall, "An Educational Intervention to Support Caregivers of Elders with Dementia," *American Journal of Alzheimer's Disease & Other Dementias* 23, no. 3 (2008): 233–41.

17. Joseph E. Gaugler, Shannon E. Jarrott, Steven H. Zarit, Mary-Ann Parris Stephens, Aloen Townsend, and Rick Greene, "Adult Day Service Use and Reductions in Caregiving Hours: Effects on Stress and Psychological Well-Being for Dementia Caregivers," *International Journal of Geriatric Psychiatry* 18, no. 1 (2003): 55–62.

18. Karen Helena Thompson and Paula Christine Fletcher, "Examining the Perceived Effects of an Adult Day Program for Individuals with Dementia and Their Caregivers: A Qualitative Investigation," *Clinical Nurse Specialist* 33, no. 1 (2019): 33–42.

19. Martin Orrell, Rob Butler, and Paul Bebbington, "Social Factors and the Outcome of Dementia," *International Journal of Geriatric Psychiatry* 15, no. 6 (2000): 515–20.

20. Gabriele Carbone, Francesca Barreca, Giovanni Mancini, Giovanni Pauletti, Veronica Salvi, Nicola Vanacore, Carla Salvitti, Fiorella Ubaldi, and Luigi Sinibaldi, "A Home Assistance Model for Dementia: Outcome

in Patients with Mild-to-Moderate Alzheimer's Disease after Three Months," *Annali dell'Istituto superiore di sanità* 49 (2013): 34–41.

21. Linda Johansson, Lennart Christensson, and Birgitta Sidenvall, "Managing Mealtime Tasks: Told by Persons with Dementia," *Journal of Clinical Nursing* 20, nos. 17–18 (2011): 2552–62.

22. Melissa J. Armstrong and Slande Alliance, "Virtual Support Groups for Informal Caregivers of Individuals with Dementia: A Scoping Review," *Alzheimer Disease and Associated Disorders* 33, no. 4 (2019): 362–69.

23. Ling-Yu Chien, Hsin Chu, Jong-Long Guo, Yuan-Mei Liao, Lu-I Chang, Chiung-Hua Chen, and Kuei-Ru Chou, "Caregiver Support Groups in Patients with Dementia: A Meta-Analysis," *International Journal of Geriatric Psychiatry* 26, no. 10 (2011): 1089–98.

24. Kenneth W. Hepburn, Jane Tornatore, Bruce Center, and Sharon W. Ostwald, "Dementia Family Caregiver Training: Affecting Beliefs about Caregiving and Caregiver Outcomes," *Journal of the American Geriatrics Society* 49, no. 4 (2001): 450–57.

25. Lia Sousa, Carlos Sequeira, Carme Ferré-Grau, Pedro Neves, and Mar Lleixà-Fortuño, "Training Programmes for Family Caregivers of People with Dementia Living at Home: Integrative Review," *Journal of Clinical Nursing* 25, nos. 19–20 (2016): 2757–67.

26. Henry Brodaty and Marika Donkin, "Family Caregivers of People with Dementia," *Dialogues in Clinical Neuroscience* (2022): DOI: 10.31887/DCNS.2009.11.2/hbrodaty.

27. Nancy L. Mace and Peter V. Rabins, *The 36-Hour Day: A Family Guide to Caring for People Who Have Alzheimer Disease, Related Dementias, and Memory Loss,* 5th ed. (Baltimore, MD: Johns Hopkins University Press, 2011).

28. Margot E. Kurtz, J. C. Kurtz, Charles W. Given, and Barbara Given, "A Randomized, Controlled Trial of a Patient/Caregiver Symptom Control Intervention: Effects on Depressive Symptomatology of Caregivers of Cancer Patients," *Journal of Pain and Symptom Management* 30, no. 2 (2005): 112–22.

29. Teresa M. Edenfield and James A. Blumenthal, "Exercise and Stress Reduction," in *The Handbook of Stress Science*, edited by Richard J. Contrada and Andrew Baum, pp. 301–20 (New York: Springer, 2011).

30. Chenlu Gao, Nikita Y. Chapagain, and Michael K. Scullin, "Sleep Duration and Sleep Quality in Caregivers of Patients with Dementia: A Systematic Review and Meta-Analysis," *JAMA Network Open* 2, no. 8 (2019): e199891.

31. Cristiano L. Guarana, Christopher M. Barnes, and Wei Jee Ong, "The Effects of Blue-Light Filtration on Sleep and Work Outcomes," *Journal of Applied Psychology* 106, no. 5 (2021): 784.

CHAPTER 2

1. Kenneth E. Foote and Maoz Azaryahu, "Toward a Geography of Memory: Geographical Dimensions of Public Memory and Commemoration," *Journal of Political and Military Sociology* (2007): 125–44.

2. Justine McGovern, "Capturing the Significance of Place in the Lived Experience of Dementia," *Qualitative Social Work* 16, no. 5 (2017): 664–79.

3. Ray Oldenburg, "The Character of Third Places," in *The Great Good Place*, pp. 20–42 (Cambridge, MA: Da Capo, 1999).

4. Jacinta Robertson, David Evans, and Tim Horsnell, "Side by Side: A Workplace Engagement Program for People with Younger Onset Dementia," *Dementia* 12, no. 5 (2013): 666–74.

5. Paul A. Rodgers, "Designing Work with People Living with Dementia: Reflecting on a Decade of Research," *International Journal of Environmental Research and Public Health* 18, no. 22 (2021): 11742.

6. Oldenburg, "The Character of Third Places."

7. Jiska Cohen-Mansfield and Perla Werner, "Environmental Influences on Agitation: An Integrative Summary of an Observational Study," *American Journal of Alzheimer's Care and Related Disorders & Research* 10, no. 1 (1995): 32–39.

8. Susan Pinker, *The Village Effect: How Face-to-Face Contact Can Make Us Healthier and Happier* (Toronto, ON: Vintage Books Canada, 2015).

9. Wei Qiao Qiu, Michael Dean, Timothy Liu, Linda George, Margery Gann, Joshua Cohen, and Martha L. Bruce, "Physical and Mental Health of Homebound Older Adults: An Overlooked Population," *Journal of the American Geriatrics Society* 58, no. 12 (2010): 2423–28.

10. Laura L. Carstensen and Christine R. Hartel, *When I'm 64* (Washington, DC: The National Academies Press, 2006).

11. Oldenburg, "The Character of Third Places."

12. D. Doran, A. Edgley, and T. Stickley, "'You Feel Like the One that Got Left Behind': A Narrative Inquiry into the Friendships of People Who Have Endured Mental Health Difficulties," *Perspectives in Public Health* (2021): 17579139211035161.

13. Susan L. Hutchinson and Karen A. Gallant, "Can Senior Centres Be Contexts for Aging in Third Places," *Journal of Leisure Research* 48, no. 1 (2016): 50–68.

14. Kirsty M. Patterson, Chris Clarke, Emma L. Wolverson, and Esme D. Moniz-Cook, "Through the Eyes of Others: The Social Experiences of People with Dementia: A Systematic Literature Review and Synthesis," *International Psychogeriatrics* 30, no. 6 (2018): 791–805.

15. Jan Dougherty, *Travel Well with Dementia: Essential Tips to Enjoy the Journey* (Pennsauken, NJ: BookBaby, 2019).

CHAPTER 3

1. Esther M. Sternberg, *Healing Spaces: The Science of Place and Well-Being* (Cambridge, MA: Harvard University Press, 2010).

2. J. M. Leger, R. Moulias, B. Vellas, J. C. Monfort, P. Chapuy, P. Robert, S. Knellesen, and D. Gerard, "Causes and Consequences of Elderly's Agitated and Aggressive Behavior," *L'encephale* 26, no. 1 (2000): 32–43.

3. Hyochol Ahn and Ann Horgas, "The Relationship between Pain and Disruptive Behaviors in Nursing Home Resident with Dementia," *BMC Geriatrics* 13, no. 1 (2013): 1–7.

4. Changbae Lee, Sang Cheol Lee, Yeon Seob Shin, Sangwoo Park, Ki Bum Won, Soe Hee Ann, and Eun Jae Ko, "Severity, Progress, and Related Factors of Mood Disorders in Patients with Coronary Artery Disease: A Retrospective Study," In *Healthcare* 8, no. 4 (2020): 568.

5. Barbara Huelat and Sharon T. Pochron, "Stress in the Volunteer Caregiver: Human-Centric Technology Can Support Both Caregivers and People with Dementia," *Medicina* 56, no. 6 (2020): 257.

6. Robyn Gillespie, Judy Mullan, and Lindsey Harrison, "Managing Medications: The Role of Informal Caregivers of Older Adults and People Living with Dementia: A Review of the Literature," *Journal of Clinical Nursing* 23, no. 23–24 (2014): 3296–308.

7. Rebecka Fleetwood-Smith, Victoria Tischler, and Deirdre Robson, "Using Creative, Sensory and Embodied Research Methods When Working with People with Dementia: A Method Story," *Arts & Health* 14, no. 3 (2022): 263–79.

8. Erik Koomen, Craig S. Webster, David Konrad, Johannes G. van der Hoeven, Thomas Best, Jozef Kesecioglu, Diederik AMPJ Gommers, Willem B. de Vries, and Teus H. Kappen, "Reducing Medical Device Alarms by an Order of Magnitude: A Human Factors Approach," *Anaesthesia and Intensive Care* 49, no. 1 (2021): 52–61.

9. Huelat and Pochron, "Stress in the Volunteer Caregiver."

10. B. Sutor, T. A. Rummans, and G. E. Smith, "Assessment and Management of Behavioral Disturbances in Nursing Home Patients with Dementia," *Mayo Clin Proc.* 76, no. 5 (2001): 540–50.

11. Ibid.

12. Ibid.

13. Ibid.

14. Ibid.

15. Vivian Isaac, Abraham Kuot, Mohammad Hamiduzzaman, Edward Strivens, and Jennene Greenhill, "The Outcomes of a Person-Centered, Non-Pharmacological Intervention in Reducing Agitation in Residents with Dementia in Australian Rural Nursing Homes," *BMC Geriatrics* 21, no. 1 (2021): 1–11.

16. Paula Piirainen, Hanna-Mari Pesonen, Helvi Kyngäs, and Satu Elo, "Challenging Situations and Competence of Nursing Staff in Nursing Homes for Older People with Dementia," *International Journal of Older People Nursing* 16, no. 5 (2021): e12384.

17. Luke Emrich-Mills, Vaisakh Puthusseryppady, and Michael Hornberger, "Effectiveness of Interventions for Preventing People with Dementia Exiting or Getting Lost," *The Gerontologist* 61, no. 3 (2021): e48–60.

18. Ipsit V. Vahia, Zachary Kabelac, Chen-Yu Hsu, Brent P. Forester, Patrick Monette, Rose May, Katherine Hobbs, Usman Munir, Kreshnik Hoti, and Dina Katabi, "Radio Signal Sensing and Signal Processing to Monitor Behavioral Symptoms in Dementia: A Case Study," *The American Journal of Geriatric Psychiatry* 28, no. 8 (2020): 820–25.

19. Melinda La Garce, "Daylight Interventions and Alzheimer's Behaviors: A Twelve-Month Study," *Journal of Architectural and Planning Research* (2004): 257–69.

20. Adebusola A. Adekoya and Lorna Guse, "Wandering Behavior from the Perspectives of Older Adults with Mild to Moderate Dementia in Long-Term Care," *Research in Gerontological Nursing* 12, no. 5 (2019): 239–47.

21. Jose Gines Gimenez Manuel, Juan Carlos Augusto, and Jill Stewart, "AnAbEL: Towards Empowering People Living with Dementia in Ambient Assisted Living," *Universal Access in the Information Society* (2020): 1–20.

CHAPTER 4

1. Habib Chaudhury and Graham D. Rowles, "Between the Shores of Recollection and Imagination: Self, Aging, and Home," *Home and Identity in Late Life: International Perspectives* (2005): 3–18.

2. Maï-Carmen Requena-Komuro, Charles R. Marshall, Rebecca L. Bond, Lucy L. Russell, Caroline Greaves, Katrina M. Moore, Jennifer L. Agustus, et al., "Altered Time Awareness in Dementia," *Frontiers in Neurology* 11 (2020): 291.

3. Ann Forsyth and Jennifer Molinsky, "What Is Aging in Place? Confusions and Contradictions," *Housing Policy Debate* 31, no. 2 (2021): 181–96.

4. Natalie Rosel, "Aging in Place: Knowing Where You Are," *The International Journal of Aging and Human Development* 57, no. 1 (2003): 77–90.

5. Esther Iecovich, "Aging in Place: From Theory to Practice," *Anthropological Notebooks* 20, no. 1 (2014).

6. Linn Hege Førsund, Ellen Karine Grov, Anne-Sofie Helvik, Lene Kristine Juvet, Kirsti Skovdahl, and Siren Eriksen, "The Experience of Lived Space in Persons with Dementia: A Systematic Meta-Synthesis," *BMC Geriatrics* 18, no. 1 (2018): 1–27.

7. Wenjin Wang and Zhipeng Lu, "Influences of Physical Environmental Cues on People with Dementia: A Scoping Review," *Journal of Applied Gerontology* 41, no. 4 (2022): 1209–21.

8. Ibid.

9. Li Feng Tan and Santhosh Seetharaman, "Preventing the Spread of COVID-19 to Nursing Homes: Experience from a Singapore Geriatric Centre," *Journal of the American Geriatrics Society* 68, no. 5 (2020): 942.

10. Joseph E. Gaugler, Mary S. Mittelman, Kenneth Hepburn, and Robert Newcomer, "Predictors of Change in Caregiver Burden and Depressive

Symptoms Following Nursing Home Admission," *Psychology and Aging* 24, no. 2 (2009): 385.

CHAPTER 5

1. Eileen B. Malone and Barbara A. Dellinger, "Furniture Design Features and Healthcare Outcomes" (Concord, CA: The Center for Health Design, 2011).

2. Julian C. Hughes, *How We Think about Dementia: Personhood, Rights, Ethics, the Arts and What They Mean for Care* (London: Jessica Kingsley Publishers, 2014).

3. Joanna Lenham, "Colour, Contrast and Comfort: Interior Design in Dementia," *Nursing and Residential Care* 15, no. 9 (2013): 616–18.

4. I. Mebane-Sims, "Alzheimer's Association, 2018 Alzheimer's Disease Facts and Figures," *Alzheimer's Dementia* 14, no. 3 (2018): 367–429.

5. Lucas A. Keefer, Mark J. Landau, Zachary K. Rothschild, and Daniel Sullivan, "Attachment to Objects as Compensation for Close Others' Perceived Unreliability," *Journal of Experimental Social Psychology* 48, no. 4 (2012): 912–17.

6. Gowri Betrabet Gulwadi, "Establishing Continuity of Self-Memory Boxes in Dementia Facilities for Older Adults: Their Use and Usefulness," *Journal of Housing for the Elderly* 27, nos. 1–2 (2013): 105–19.

7. Ponnusamy Subramaniam and Bob Woods, "The Impact of Individual Reminiscence Therapy for People with Dementia: Systematic Review," *Expert Review of Neurotherapeutics* 12, no. 5 (2012): 545–55.

8. Cameron J. Camp, "Origins of Montessori Programming for Dementia," *Non-Pharmacological Therapies in Dementia* 1, no. 2 (2010): 163.

9. Kala Chinnaswamy, Dominic M. DeMarco, and George T. Grossberg, "Doll Therapy in Dementia: Facts and Controversies," *Annals of Clinical Psychiatry* 33 (2021): 58–66.

10. John Zeisel, Michael J. Skrajner, Evan B. Zeisel, Miranda Noelle Wilson, and Chris Gage, "Scripted-IMPROV: Interactive Improvisational Drama with Persons with Dementia—Effects on Engagement, Affect, Depression, and Quality of Life," *American Journal of Alzheimer's Disease and Other Dementias*® 33, no. 4 (2018): 232–41.

CHAPTER 6

1. Miranda M. Lim, Jason R. Gerstner, and David M. Holtzman, "The Sleep–Wake Cycle and Alzheimer's Disease: What Do We Know?" *Neurodegenerative Disease Management* 4, no. 5 (2014): 351–62.

2. Lim, Gerstner, and Holtzman, "The Sleep–Wake Cycle and Alzheimer's Disease: What Do We Know?"

3. Suzanne Hood and Shimon Amir, "Neurodegeneration and the Circadian Clock," *Frontiers in Aging Neuroscience* 9 (2017): 170.

4. Lim, Gerstner, and Holtzman, "The Sleep–Wake Cycle and Alzheimer's Disease: What Do We Know?"

5. Rachael M. Kelly, Ultan Healy, Seamus Sreenan, John H. McDermott, and Andrew N. Coogan, "Clocks in the Clinic: Circadian Rhythms in Health and Disease," *Postgraduate Medical Journal* 94, no. 1117 (2018): 653–58.

6. Else Lykkeslet, Eva Gjengedal, Torill Skrondal, and May-Britt Storjord, "Sensory Stimulation—A Way of Creating Mutual Relations in Dementia Care," *International Journal of Qualitative Studies on Health and Well-Being* 9, no. 1 (2014): 23888.

7. Judith M. Torrington and P. R. Tregenza, "Lighting for People with Dementia," *Lighting Research and Technology* 39, no. 1 (2007): 81–97.

8. Elizabeth C. Brawley, *Designing for Alzheimer's Disease: Strategies for Creating Better Care Environments* (New York: Wiley & Sons, 1997).

9. Han van der Rhee, Esther de Vries, Claudia Coomans, Piet van de Velde, and Jan W. Coebergh, "Sunlight: For Better or for Worse? A Review of

Positive and Negative Effects of Sun Exposure," *Cancer Research Frontiers* 2, no. 2 (2016): 156–83.

10. Michael D. White, Sonia Ancoli-Israel, and Richard R. Wilson, "Senior Living Environments: Evidence-Based Lighting Design Strategies," *HERD: Health Environments Research and Design Journal* 7, no. 1 (2013): 60–78.

11. Paweł Korpal and Katarzyna Jankowiak, "On the Potential Impact of Directionality on Emotion Processing in Interpreting," *Onomázein: Revista de lingüística, filología y traducción de la Pontificia Universidad Católica de Chile* 8 (2021): 43–60.

12. Shariful Shikder, Monjur Mourshed, and Andrew Price, "Therapeutic Lighting Design for the Elderly: A Review," *Perspectives in Public Health* 132, no. 6 (2012): 282–91.

13. Alistair Burns, Harry Allen, Barbara Tomenson, Debbie Duignan, and Jane Byrne, "Bright Light Therapy for Agitation in Dementia: A Randomized Controlled Trial," *International Psychogeriatrics* 21, no. 4 (2009): 711–21.

14. Oludamilola Salami, Constantine Lyketsos, and Vani Rao, "Treatment of Sleep Disturbance in Alzheimer's Dementia," *International Journal of Geriatric Psychiatry* 26, no. 8 (2011): 771–82.

15. Nuria Cibeira, Ana Maseda, Laura Lorenzo-López, Isabel González-Abraldes, Rocío López-López, José L. Rodríguez-Villamil, and José C. Millán-Calenti, "Bright Light Therapy in Older Adults with Moderate to Very Severe Dementia: Immediate Effects on Behavior, Mood, and Physiological Parameters," in *Healthcare* 9, no. 8 (2021): 1065.

16. Jun Song Isaac Tan, Ling Jie Cheng, Ee Yuee Chan, Ying Lau, and Siew Tiang Lau, "Light Therapy for Sleep Disturbances in Older Adults with Dementia: A Systematic Review, Meta-Analysis, and Meta-Regression," *Sleep Medicine* (2022).

17. Chanung Wang and David M. Holtzman, "Bidirectional Relationship between Sleep and Alzheimer's Disease: Role of Amyloid, Tau, and Other Factors," *Neuropsychopharmacology* 45, no. 1 (2020): 104–20.

CHAPTER 7

1. Ben Street, *How to Enjoy Art: A Guide for Everyone* (New Haven, CT: Yale University Press, 2021).

2. Banu Manav, "A Research on Light-Color Perception: Can Visual Images Be Used Instead of 1/1 Model Study for Space Perception?" *Psychology* 4, no. 9 (2013): 711.

3. Carl J. Bassi, Kenneth Solomon, and Dwayne Young, "Vision in Aging and Dementia," *Optometry and Vision Science: Official Publication of the American Academy of Optometry* 70, no. 10 (1993): 809–13.

4. Johannes Itten, *The Elements of Color*, vol. 4 (Hoboken, NJ: John Wiley & Sons, 1970).

5. Banu Manav, "Color-Emotion Associations and Color Preferences: A Case Study for Residences," *Color Research & Application: Endorsed by Inter-Society Color Council, The Colour Group (Great Britain), Canadian Society for Color, Color Science Association of Japan, Dutch Society for the Study of Color, The Swedish Colour Centre Foundation, Colour Society of Australia, Centre Français de la Couleur* 32, no. 2 (2007): 144–50.

6. Manav, "Color-Emotion Associations and Color Preferences."

7. Andrew J. Elliot, Markus A. Maier, Arlen C. Moller, Ron Friedman, and Jörg Meinhardt, "Color and Psychological Functioning: The Effect of Red on Performance Attainment," *Journal of Experimental Psychology: General* 136, no. 1 (2007): 154.

8. Jain Malkin, *Hospital Interior Architecture: Creating Healing Environments for Special Patient Populations* (Washington, DC: Van Nostrand Reinhold Company, 1992).

9. Sheila J. Bosch, Rosalyn Cama, Eve Edelstein, and Jain Malkin, "The Application of Color in Healthcare Settings," *The Center for Health Design* (2012): 1–78.

10. Andrew J. Elliot, Markus A. Maier, Arlen C. Moller, Ron Friedman, and Jörg Meinhardt, "Color and Psychological Functioning: The Effect of Red on Performance Attainment," *Journal of Experimental Psychology: General* 136, no. 1 (2007): 154.

11. Ibid.

12. Ibid.

13. Barbara J. Huelat, "The Wisdom of Biophilia—Nature in Healing Environments," *Journal of Green Building* 3, no. 3 (2008): 23–35.

14. Bosch, Cama, Edelstein, and Malkin, "The Application of Color in Healthcare Settings."

15. Ibid.

16. Ibid.

17. Ibid.

18. Margaret P. Calkins, "Using Color as Therapeutic Tool," *Ideas Institute Publications. Publications Sites of Ideas Institute* (2010) (online) http://www.ideasinstitute.org/article_021103_b.asp (accessed on February 9, 2018).

19. Michelangelo Stanzani Maserati, Micaela Mitolo, Federica Medici, Renato D'Onofrio, Federico Oppi, Roberto Poda, Maddalena De Matteis, et al., "Color Choice Preference in Cognitively Impaired Patients: A Look Inside Alzheimer's Disease through the Use of Lüscher Color Diagnostic," *Frontiers in Psychology* 10 (2019): 1951.

20. John Zeisel, *I'm Still Here: A Breakthrough Approach to Understanding Someone Living with Alzheimer's* (New York: Penguin, 2009).

21. Qiu-Yue Wang and Dong-Mei Li, "Advances in Art Therapy for Patients with Dementia," *Chinese Nursing Research* 3, no. 3 (2016): 105–8.

CHAPTER 8

1. Thomas T. H. Wan and Bing Long Wang, "An Integrated Social and Behavioral System Approach to Evaluation of Healthcare Information Technology for Polychronic Conditions," *Journal of Integrated Design and Process Science* 25, nos. 3–4 (2021): 1–14.

2. Barbara Huelat and Sharon T. Pochron, "Stress in the Volunteer Caregiver: Human-Centric Technology Can Support Both Caregivers and People with Dementia," *Medicina* 56, no. 6 (2020): 257.

3. Allison H. Burfield, Thomas T. H. Wan, Mary Lou Sole, and James W. Cooper, "A Study of Longitudinal Data Examining Concomitance of Pain and Cognition in an Elderly Long-Term Care Population," *Journal of Pain Research* 5 (2012): 61–70. doi: 10.2147/JPR.S29655.

4. Burfield et al., "A Study of Longitudinal Data Examining Concomitance of Pain and Cognition in an Elderly Long-Term Care Population."

5. Wan and Wang, "An Integrated Social and Behavioral System Approach to Evaluation of Healthcare Information Technology for Polychronic Conditions."

6. Lora Appel, Suad Ali, Tanya Narag, Krystyna Mozeson, Zain Pasat, Ani Orchanian-Cheff, and Jennifer L. Campos, "Virtual Reality to Promote Wellbeing in Persons with Dementia: A Scoping Review," *Journal of Rehabilitation and Assistive Technologies Engineering* 8 (2021): 20556683211053952.

7. Hui-Min Chiu, Mei-Chi Hsu, and Wen-Chen Ouyang, "Effects of Incorporating Virtual Reality Training Intervention into Health Care on Cognitive Function and Wellbeing in Older Adults with Cognitive Impairment: A Randomized Controlled Trial," *International Journal of Human-Computer Studies* 170 (2023): 102957.

CHAPTER 9

1. Edward O. Wilson, *Biophilia* (Boston: Harvard University Press, 1986).

2. Stephen R. Kellert, "Dimensions, Elements, and Attributes of Biophilic Design," *Biophilic Design: The Theory, Science, and Practice of Bringing Buildings to Life* (2008): 3–19.

3. Caoimhe Twohig-Bennett and Andy Jones, "The Health Benefits of the Great Outdoors: A Systematic Review and Meta-Analysis of Greenspace Exposure and Health Outcomes," *Environmental Research* 166 (2018): 628–37.

4. Victoria Houlden, Scott Weich, João Porto de Albuquerque, Stephen Jarvis, and Karen Rees, "The Relationship Between Greenspace and the Mental Wellbeing of Adults: A Systematic Review," *PLOS ONE* 13, no. 9 (2018): e0203000.

5. He-Ying Hu, Ya-Hui Ma, Yue-Ting Deng, Ya-Nan Ou, Wei Cheng, Jian-Feng Feng, Lan Tan, and Jin-Tai Yu, "Residential Greenness and Risk of Incident Dementia: A Prospective Study of 375,342 Participants," *Environmental Research* 216 (2023): 114703.

6. Marcia P. Jimenez, Elise G. Elliott, Nicole V. DeVille, Francine Laden, Jaime E. Hart, Jennifer Weuve, Francine Grodstein, and Peter James, "Residential Green Space and Cognitive Function in a Large Cohort of Middle-Aged Women," *JAMA Network Open* 5, no. 4 (2022): e229306–e229306.

7. Takemi Sugiyama, Alison Carver, Masaaki Sugiyama, Alanna Lorenzon, and Tanya E. Davison, "Views of Greenery and Psychological Well-Being in Residential Aged Care Facilities: Longitudinal Associations," *HERD: Health Environments Research & Design Journal* 15, no. 2 (2022): 219–32.

8. Matthew H. E. M. Browning, Kangjae Lee, and Kathleen L. Wolf, "Tree Cover Shows an Inverse Relationship with Depressive Symptoms in Elderly Residents Living in US Nursing Homes," *Urban Forestry & Urban Greening* 41 (2019): 23–32.

9. Alison Carver, Alanna Lorenzon, Jenny Veitch, Ashley Macleod, and Takemi Sugiyama, "Is Greenery Associated with Mental Health among Residents of Aged Care Facilities? A Systematic Search and Narrative Review," *Aging and Mental Health* 24, no. 1 (2020): 1–7.

10. Tianyu Zhao, Iana Markevych, Dorota Buczyłowska, Marcel Romanos, and Joachim Heinrich, "When Green Enters a Room: A Scoping Review of Epidemiological Studies on Indoor Plants and Mental Health," *Environmental Research* (2022): 114715.

11. Mathew P. White, Ian Alcock, James Grellier, Benedict W. Wheeler, Terry Hartig, Sara L. Warber, Angie Bone, Michael H. Depledge, and Lora E. Fleming, "Spending at Least 120 Minutes a Week in Nature Is Associated with Good Health and Wellbeing," *Scientific Reports* 9, no. 1 (2019): 1–11.

12. Barbara J. Huelat, *Healing Environments: What's the Proof?* (Novi, MI: Medezyn, 2007).

13. Amjad Hasan Bazzari and Firas Hasan Bazzari, "Medicinal Plants for Alzheimer's Disease: An Updated Review," *Journal of Medicinal Plants* 6, no. 2 (2018): 81–85.

14. Kellert, "Dimensions, Elements, and Attributes of Biophilic Design."

15. J. Warmuth and J. Joseph, "The Effects of a Waterfall on the Systolic Blood Pressure of Individuals with Dementia," *Healthcare Design* (2008).

16. Kellert, "Dimensions, Elements, and Attributes of Biophilic Design."

17. Alan M. Beck, "The Biology of the Human–Animal Bond," *Animal Frontiers* 4, no. 3 (2014): 32–36.

18. Kent W. Myers, Dina Capek, Holly Shill, and Marwan Sabbagh, "Aquatic Therapy and Alzheimer's Disease," *Annals of Long-Term Care* 21, no. 5 (2013): 36–41.

CHAPTER 10

1. Esther M. Sternberg, *The Balance Within: The Science Connecting Health and Emotions* (New York: Macmillan, 2001).

2. Masahiko Fujii, James P. Butler, and Hidetada Sasaki, "Emotional Function in Dementia Patients," *Psychogeriatrics* 14, no. 3 (2014): 202–9.

3. Sternberg, *The Balance Within*.

4. Catherine Rouby, Arnaud Fournel, and Moustafa Bensafi, "The Role of the Senses in Emotion," in *Emotion Measurement*, edited by Herbert L. Meiselman, pp. 65–81 (Cambridge, UK: Woodhead Publishing, 2016).

5. Chin-Mei Liu and Charles Tzu-Chi Lee, "Association of Hearing Loss with Dementia," *JAMA Network Open* 2, no. 7 (2019): e198112.

6. Magda Bucholc, Sarah Bauermeister, Daman Kaur, Paula L. McClean, and Stephen Todd, "The Impact of Hearing Impairment and Hearing Aid Use on Progression to Mild Cognitive Impairment in Cognitively Healthy Adults: An Observational Cohort Study," *Alzheimer's and Dementia: Translational Research and Clinical Interventions* 8, no. 1 (2022): e12248.

7. Amee Baird and Séverine Samson, "Music and Dementia," *Progress in Brain Research* 217 (2015): 207–35.

8. Rebecca Dahms, Cornelia Eicher, Marten Haesner, and Ursula Mueller-Werdan, "Influence of Music Therapy and Music-Based Interventions on Dementia: A Pilot Study," *Journal of Music Therapy* 58, no. 3 (2021): e12–36.

9. Ibid.

10. Yu Wang, Kokoro Shirai, Tetsuya Ohira, Mayumi Hirosaki, Naoki Kondo, Kenji Takeuchi, Chikae Yamaguchi, et al., "Occasions for Laughter and Dementia Risk: Findings from a Six-Year Cohort Study," *Geriatrics and Gerontology International* (2022).

11. Areum Han, Mark E. Kunik, and Amber Richardson, "Compassionate Touch® Delivered by Long-Term Care Staff for Residents with Dementia: Preliminary Results," *Journal of Social Service Research* 46, no. 5 (2020): 685–92.

12. Diane Ackerman, *A Natural History of the Senses* (New York: Vintage, 1991).

13. Lee Dunn, "Theories of Learning," *Learning and Teaching Briefing Papers Series* 3 (2002).

14. Jenny C. C. Chung, Claudia K. Y. Lai, and Cochrane Dementia and Cognitive Improvement Group, "Snoezelen for Dementia," *Cochrane Database of Systematic Reviews* no. 4 (2002).

Index